SMOOTH AND SATISFYING:

Chef Vita's Guide To Making Nutritious Pureed Meals For Seniors,

Chef Vita

Table of Contents

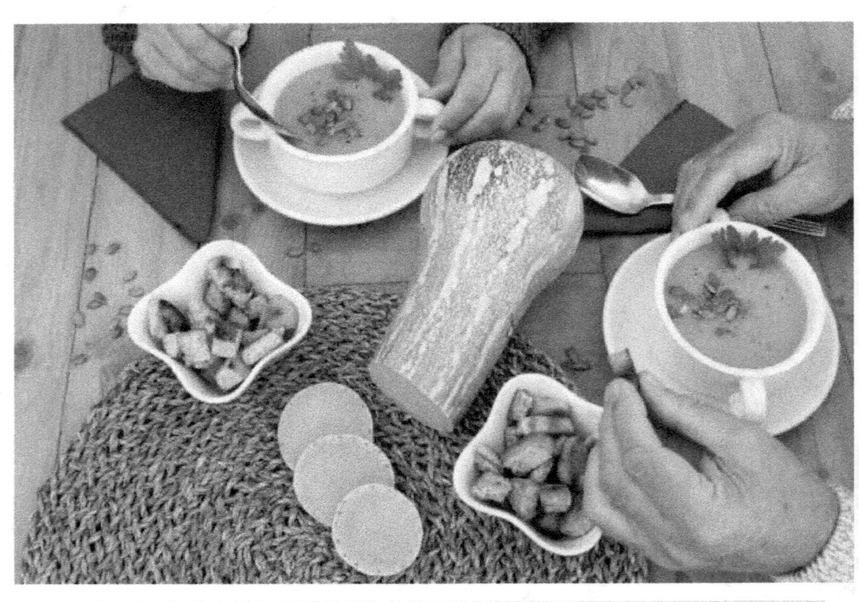

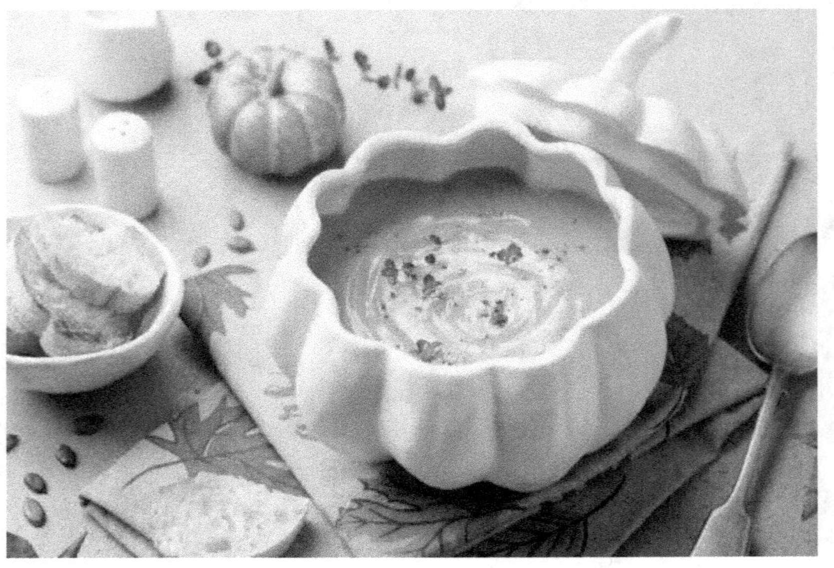

Introduction

Welcome to Chef Vita's Recipes for Seniors: Healthy Pureed Meals! We go over all you need to know about preparing delicious and nutritious pureed meals for the elderly in this detailed tutorial.

We'll start by discussing the importance of pureed meals for elderly people with dysphagia and other medical issues. We also talk about the risks associated with dysphagia, such as choking, dehydration, aspiration pneumonia, and malnutrition.

But don't panic, you can make pureed meals that are delightful and nourishing if you use the correct methods and tools. We'll go into food pureeing techniques and the tools required for the best outcomes.

Of course, we also need to remember the ingredients. We'll present you with some delectable pureed diet recipes to get you started as well as advice on how to select high-quality products that are ideal for pureeing.

With the help of Chef Vita's Guide to Making Nutritious Pureed Meals for Seniors, you'll have all the information and resources required to make scrumptious and nutritious pureed meals for older family members or clients.

As our loved ones age, dental problems, illnesses, or other health conditions may make it difficult for them to chew and swallow food. Food that has been pureed is a great alternative for people who have trouble eating solid food. For elderly people who may find it more difficult to obtain the nutrition they require, it may be simpler to swallow, digest, and give important nutrients.

We'll look at the advantages of homemade pureed food for seniors in this tutorial, as well as how to cook wholesome meals. We'll go through the necessary supplies for pureeing, the many kinds of pureed food, and the numerous methods for making pureed meals. Additionally, we'll provide recipes for breakfast, lunch, dinner, snacks, and dessert, as well as special diet recipes for people who have particular dietary requirements. Finally, we'll go over meal preparation and storage to make pureed meals both wholesome and practical.

By the time you finish reading this book, you'll know more about pureed food and how to cook wholesome meals that your family will appreciate. So let's get going!

It's crucial to recognize the value of pureed meals since they can help elders live better lives. Many elderly people experience malnutrition for a variety of reasons, including loss of appetite, problems swallowing or chewing, and digestive problems. Healthy pureed foods can give senior citizens the nutrition they require to maintain their health and level of energy.

Additionally, homemade pureed food is a superior substitute for prepared meals from the store. Commercially prepared pureed food frequently lacks flavor and nutrients and may contain additives or preservatives that are bad for an elderly person's health. You have complete control over the ingredients and can meet particular dietary requirements by making handmade pureed meals.

It can be intimidating to prepare pureed food for elders, but with the correct equipment, methods, and recipes, it can be a satisfying experience for both the caregiver and the senior. It enables you to ensure that your loved ones enjoy their meals while still giving them the nutrients they require.

We'll provide you with practical advice and pointers throughout this manual to make preparing pureed meals for senior citizens easier. We'll walk you through the process of preparing nourishing and delectable pureed meals, from comprehending the many kinds of pureed food to giving you scrumptious recipes and meal-planning advice.

Let's explore the world of senior pureed food together!

It's critical to comprehend what pureed food is and why it's crucial for seniors before talking about the various kinds of pureed food and their advantages.

Food that has been mashed or blended to achieve a smooth, lump-free consistency is referred to as pureed food. Food that has been pureed is the perfect texture for senior citizens who have trouble chewing or swallowing since it facilitates digestion.

Consuming solid meals can be difficult and uncomfortable for seniors who have tooth problems, diseases, or other health conditions. They can enjoy a variety of nutritious meals with pureed food without the discomfort and challenge of eating solid food.

Additionally, pureed food can aid in preventing malnutrition, a problem that affects many elderly people. Over 10% of senior citizens worldwide suffer from malnutrition, according to the World Health Organization (WHO). Seniors can easily get the nutrients they require to preserve their health and welfare by serving them pureed cuisine.

Let's examine the many kinds of pureed food and their advantages now that we are aware of what they are and how important they are.

- Description Of Dysphagia?

Dysphagia is a term used in medicine to describe problems with swallowing food, liquids, or saliva. Although it can happen at any age, older persons are more likely to experience it because of aging-related changes to the muscles and nerves involved in swallowing. Dysphagia can range from a minor discomfort to a serious disorder that makes it impossible for a person to drink or eat enough to stay healthy. It can be brought on by many conditions, including anatomical abnormalities like tumors or esophageal constriction, as well as neurological conditions like Parkinson's disease or stroke. Dysphagia should be diagnosed and treated right away since it can cause major health issues like choking, aspiration pneumonia, malnutrition, and dehydration.

- The Benefits Of Pureed Food For Elderly People With Dysphagia

For elderly people with dysphagia, pureed food is crucial because it offers a secure and comfortable alternative to solid food, which can be challenging to swallow and a choking hazard. Seniors frequently suffer from dysphagia, a disorder that impairs their capacity to securely swallow food or liquids. It may be brought on by several ailments, such as cancer, neurological problems, stroke, head or neck injuries, or other illnesses.

Seniors with dysphagia can benefit from eating pureed food to help them acquire the nutrients they need to stay healthy and happy. Food is mashed or blended into a smooth, lump-free consistency that is simpler to chew and digest

when it is pureed. This lessens the possibility of
choking and aspiration, a condition where food
or liquid enters the airway rather than the
digestive tract, and can result in pneumonia and
other medical issues.

meals that have been pureed can be more
nutrient-dense than solid meals, in addition to
being a safer way to ingest food. This is so that
nutrients that might be hard to obtain in solid
meals can be broken down and released through
the pureeing process. Additionally, it can make it
simpler for seniors to digest meals and absorb
nutrients, which is crucial for people who are
malnourished or have digestive problems.

Overall, pureed food can assist seniors with
dysphagia maintain their nutritional status,
avoiding health issues, and enjoying a variety of
delectable meals without discomfort or
difficulties.

- Repercussions associated with dysphagia is this correct

Seniors who have dysphagia, or trouble swallowing, run some health risks and problems. These consist of:

1. Malnutrition: A senior may not get enough nutrients to meet their body's demands if they are unable to eat enough or have trouble swallowing. This can result in malnutrition.

2. Dehydration: Similar to malnutrition, it might be difficult to drink enough fluids, which can result in dehydration.

3. Aspiration pneumonia: Aspiration pneumonia is a potentially fatal illness that occurs when

food or liquid reaches the lungs rather than the stomach.

4. Choking: Choking, which can also be fatal, is a risk that is increased by difficulty swallowing.

It's crucial to treat dysphagia seriously and use management strategies, such as introducing pureed food into older citizens' meals. Seniors who consume pureed food are more likely to get the nourishment and fluids they require to stay healthy and help lower their risk of choking and aspiration pneumonia.

- Importance Of Nutritious Pureed Meals For Seniors

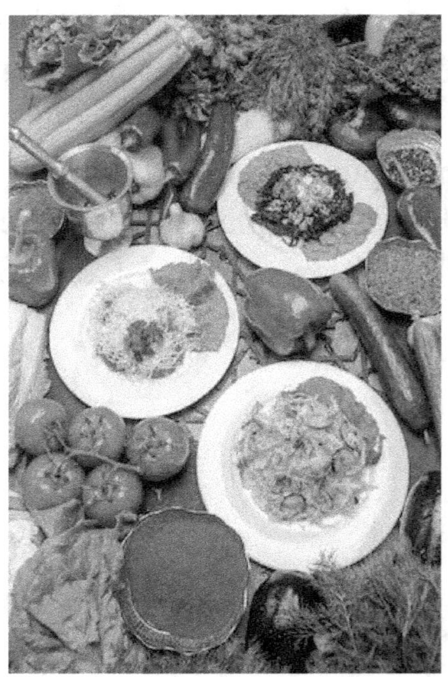

For several reasons, seniors need nourishing pureed meals. To begin with, as we age, our bodies undergo changes that can make it difficult to eat solid foods. Dental issues, a compromised sense of taste or smell, and many medical conditions can all contribute to swallowing and chewing difficulties. Pureed meals may offer seniors a variety of nutrient options that are easy to swallow and digest.

Additionally, pureed food can help in the fight against malnutrition, a major problem for the elderly. Malnutrition-related health issues, such as weakening muscles, compromised immune systems, and other illnesses, may have a detrimental impact on a senior's quality of life. By delivering pureed meals that are full of essential nutrients, caregivers can make sure that their loved ones are getting the right nutrition.

In addition to protecting seniors' autonomy and dignity, pureed food has nutritional benefits. Seniors who struggle to eat could feel embarrassed or frustrated. Children may have more control over their eating habits and enjoy meals more when meals are pureed.

Last but not least, preparing homemade pureed meals is a great way to make sure that seniors are consuming high-quality, whole foods. The nutrients in store-bought pureed meals may be lacking, and they may also contain additives or preservatives that are harmful to the health of elderly people. Caretakers can prepare full, delicious, and dietary-specific handmade pureed meals for their loved ones.

In conclusion, aging adults require nutrient-dense pureed meals. They aid in preventing malnutrition, enable seniors to maintain their independence and sense of dignity, and can be tailored to their dietary needs.

- Advantages Of Homemade Food Puree

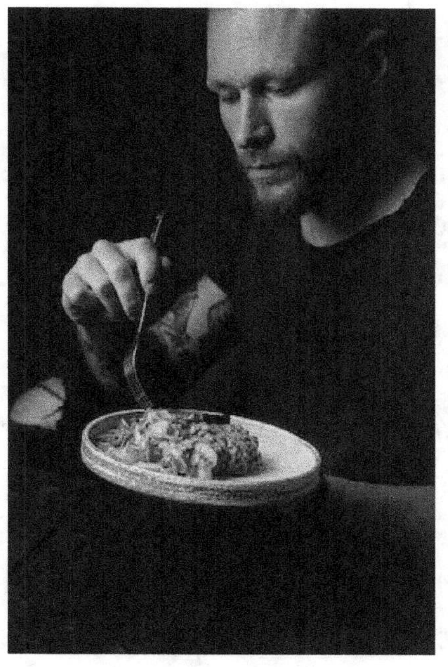

Compared to store-bought pureed foods, homemade pureed foods have numerous advantages, such as:

1. *Nutritional Value:*

Homemade pureed food often has higher levels of vital elements including vitamins, minerals, and fiber because it is produced with fresh, whole foods.

2. More affordable:
Making your own pureed food at home can be more affordable than buying ready-made pureed meals from the shop. Caregivers can reduce costs while still feeding their loved ones wholesome meals by buying fresh vegetables in bulk and cooking meals in batches.

3. Customized to Meet Specific Dietary Demands:
Homemade pureed meals can be modified to satisfy certain dietary demands. To satisfy the dietary preferences or constraints of their loved ones, caregivers can modify the texture, consistency, and components of pureed meals.

4. Better Flavor:
Homemade pureed food may have a richer flavor than selections from the grocery store.

Caregivers can prepare delightful, nutrient-dense meals by seasoning food with fresh herbs, spices, and other ingredients.

5. *No Additives or Preservatives:*
To increase the shelf life of store-bought pureed food, preservatives, and chemicals are frequently used. On the other hand, homemade pureed food may be created without any additional additives, making it a healthier alternative for elders.

6. *More Variety:*
Caregivers can provide their loved ones with a wider range of meals by producing homemade pureed food. This can help seniors stay entertained and make sure they're getting the nutrients they need from a variety of foods.

In conclusion, seniors who require pureed meals have a healthier, more affordable, and individualized choice of homemade pureed food. Caregivers can provide tasty, nourishing meals for their loved ones that are suited to their dietary requirements by doing it at home.

Chapter 1: Understanding Pureed Food

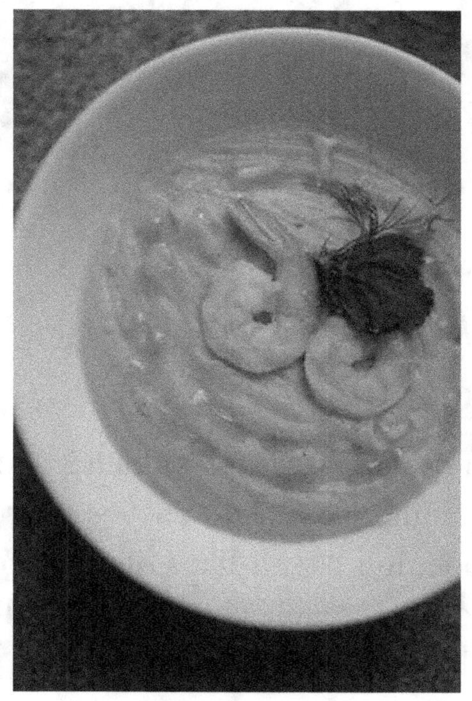

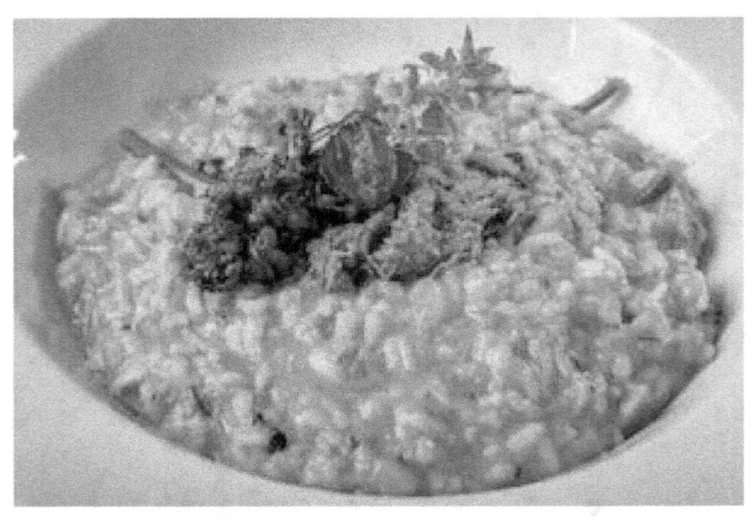

- What Is Pureed Food?

Food that has been mashed or blended to achieve a smooth, lump-free consistency is referred to as pureed food. It is a well-liked dietary choice for those who have trouble chewing or swallowing, such as elderly persons, young children, and those with particular medical issues. Fruits, vegetables, grains, meats, and dairy products can all be pureed to create a variety of dishes.

Food is often cooked before being mashed, blended, or puréed to create a smooth, uniform consistency. Pureed food may need to be thinned or thickened to attain the ideal texture depending on the person's dietary requirements. To enhance the flavor of the pureed meal, caregivers may also add seasonings or other additives.

Food that has been pureed is a valuable food choice for those who have trouble eating solid foods. It offers a secure and convenient way to eat a range of nutrient-rich foods, which can aid in preventing malnutrition and other health problems. Food that has been pureed can be prepared at home with a blender or food processor or bought ready-made from supermarkets.

It's critical to make sure the food is properly boiled and that all bones, skin, and other inedible components are removed before blending when making pureed food at home. Additionally, caregivers must consider the pureed food's texture to make sure it meets the needs of the patient. For instance, some people might like a thicker, more substantial puree, while others would need a thinner consistency.

A wide range of foods, including soups, stews, casseroles, and desserts, can be made using pureed food. Caretakers can prepare wholesome, savory pureed meals for their loved ones by experimenting with various ingredients and seasonings.

It's vital to remember that those who have trouble chewing or swallowing shouldn't limit themselves to pureed foods. To make sure that their loved ones are receiving the right nutrition, caregivers should collaborate with medical specialists to create a thorough meal plan that offers a variety of tastes and dietary alternatives.

In addition, it's critical to consider the pureed food's nutritional value. While food that has been pureed can be nutritious, if it has not been prepared properly, it may also be deficient in some nutrients. To ensure that their loved ones are receiving a balanced diet, caregivers should try to include a variety of foods in the pureed meals. This can include a variety of grains, fruits, vegetables, and proteins.

It's vital to read the label when buying prepared pureed food and to look for selections that are low in sodium, sugar, and preservatives. Before serving, caregivers should make sure the food hasn't passed its expiration date and is still fresh.

Overall, pureed food is a valuable food option for people who have trouble swallowing or chewing. Pureed food, whether produced at home or bought pre-made, may be a wholesome and delectable way to make sure your loved ones are receiving the appropriate nourishment they require. Pureed food can assist seniors and other people with particular dietary needs to enjoy a balanced and filling diet with correct preparation and nutritional consideration.

- What Justifies Seniors' Need For Pureed Food?

Seniors should consume pureed meals for a variety of reasons. People's capacity to chew and swallow food may change as they get older. This could be brought on by dental disorders, neurological conditions, or other medical conditions. Seniors can consume a range of foods safely and easily with pureed food, reducing their risk of malnutrition and other health problems.

Additionally, pureed food can assist seniors in maintaining their dignity and independence. Seniors who have trouble chewing and swallowing may find it challenging to enjoy meals and interact with others. Seniors can continue to partake in social activities and enjoy a variety of foods thanks to pureed food without having to worry about choking or other health problems.

Seniors' unique dietary requirements can be met with pureed food as well. For elderly people who have trouble chewing and swallowing, softer textures or smaller servings may be necessary. To meet these requirements and guarantee that elders are receiving the right nutrients, pureed meals can be modified.

All things considered, pureed food is a crucial food choice for seniors who have trouble chewing and swallowing. It offers a secure and convenient way to eat a range of meals, preventing malnutrition and other health problems. Caregivers can assist seniors preserve their freedom and dignity while still ensuring that they are receiving the necessary nutrition by providing pureed food as a meal choice.

- Foods That Are Pureed

A wide range of foods, including fruits, vegetables, grains, meats, and dairy products, can be pureed to create food. Here are some illustrations of various pureed food varieties:

1. **Fruit puree:** Fruits including bananas, apples, peaches, and berries are blended to a smooth, uniform consistency to create fruit puree. Fruit puree can be included in sauces, desserts, and smoothies.

2. **Vegetable puree:** To make a vegetable puree, combine steamed or cooked vegetables like carrots, sweet potatoes, broccoli, and peas in a food processor or blender and process until smooth. Vegetable puree can be served as a side dish or as the foundation for soups and stews.

3. **<u>Meat puree:</u>** To make meat puree, cooked meats like chicken, beef, or fish are blended until they have a smooth texture. In casseroles, stews, and soups, meat puree can be utilized.

4. **<u>Grain puree:</u>** To make grain puree, cook grains like rice, quinoa, or oats are blended until they have a smooth texture. A side dish or soup can be made with grain puree as the base.

5. **<u>Dairy puree:</u>** To make dairy puree, mix dairy items such as yogurt, cottage cheese, or cream cheese until they have a smooth texture. Sauces, smoothies, and desserts can all be made with dairy puree.

It is significant to remember that meals can be blended to make a variety of dishes. Caregivers can prepare wholesome and tasty meals for their loved ones by blending several pureed food varieties and adding seasonings and other ingredients.

For seniors who have particular dietary needs, there are specialist pureed food options in addition to these standard varieties of pureed foods. For instance, some pureed foods may be fortified with vitamins and minerals to add extra nourishment, while others may be created to have a reduced sodium content.

To determine which food purees work best for their loved ones, caregivers can also experiment with various textures and consistencies. While some seniors might prefer a thicker, more pudding-like consistency, others might prefer a thinner, soupier consistency.

It's also crucial to consider how pureed food is presented and colored, as this can influence a senior's appetite and satisfaction with the meal. Food that has been pureed can be improved in flavor and appeal by seasoning it with herbs, spices, and other ingredients. Adding garnishes or serving pureed food in colorful bowls can also improve its aesthetic appeal.

Seniors can choose from a wide variety of pureed foods, and caregivers can experiment with different flavors and textures to find the ones that their loved ones prefer. To assist elderly maintain their health and enjoy meals, caregivers can offer a variety of nutrient-dense and delectable pureed food options.

It's also crucial to keep in mind that some elderly people may be subject to specific dietary restrictions or medical issues that forbid them from consuming certain pureed foods. For instance, elderly people with diabetes may need to avoid sugar-rich pureed foods, while people with kidney illness may need to restrict their intake of specific types of protein.

It's crucial to work with a registered dietitian or a senior's healthcare professional to create a meal plan that accommodates any special dietary requirements or restrictions.

It's critical to make sure that pureed foods are prepared securely in addition to making sure they are nutritionally balanced and satisfy any dietary requirements. To stop the growth of dangerous bacteria, pureed foods should be handled and kept the same as ordinary food. To reduce the danger of burns or scalds, caregivers should also make sure that pureed foods are delivered at the proper temperature.

Caregivers may help elders retain their health, independence, and pleasure of meals by following these measures and offering a range of nourishing and delectable pureed food alternatives.

Finally, it's critical to keep in mind that meals should promote social interaction and enjoyment in addition to providing nutrition. Sharing meals with friends or relatives can give seniors who feel alone or cut off from their communities a sense of connection and belonging.

By including their loved ones in the meal preparation process, giving them the freedom to choose the items they want to eat, and creating a comfortable and welcoming mealtime setting, caregivers may help make mealtimes more enjoyable for their loved ones.

To sum up, pureed food can be a significant and nutrient-dense choice for seniors who have trouble swallowing or chewing. Caregivers can assist seniors in maintaining the health and enjoyment of meals by offering a range of pureed food alternatives that are nutrient-balanced, tasty, and aesthetically pleasing.

- Texture Adjustments for Various Dietary Needs

Changing the texture of pureed food might help seniors who have trouble swallowing or chewing achieve their nutritional needs. Here are a few typical texture alterations and how they can be applied to accommodate various dietary requirements:

1. **Thin Puree:** Seniors who prefer a thinner consistency or who have slight swallowing difficulties might consider this texture because it is smooth and simple to swallow. Foods can be blended with a liquid, such as broth, water, or milk, to create a thin puree.

2. **Thick Puree:** This consistency is thicker and more pudding-like, which makes it a wonderful choice for senior citizens who need a bit extra texture to help them swallow. Thin puree can be

made thicker by adding more pureed ingredients, such as mashed potatoes or beans.

3. **<u>Puree with Lumps:</u>** This texture has bits of fruit or vegetables blended into the base of the puree. Seniors who are switching from pureed food to ordinary food may find it to be a suitable alternative because it helps to develop their swallowing muscles.

4. **<u>Food that has been ground or minced into little pieces, around the size of rice grains, creates this texture.</u>** Seniors who have some trouble swallowing but can handle small portions of food may find it to be a decent option.

5. **<u>Soft Food:</u>** To get this texture, heat food until it is pliable and simple to chew. For seniors who struggle to chew due to dental or jaw issues, soft food can be an excellent option.

It's crucial to take each senior's unique dietary requirements into account when modifying the texture of pureed meals. Seniors with diabetes, for instance, might need to stay away from pureed foods with added sugars, while those with kidney problems might need to cut back on specific protein sources. It's always ideal to work with a certified dietitian or healthcare professional to create a meal plan that caters to the individual dietary requirements of each senior.

It's also crucial to keep in mind that, although texture adjustments can be beneficial for seniors who have trouble swallowing, they might not be appropriate for everyone. Some elderly people may experience more severe swallowing issues that call for a different strategy, such as a liquid or pureed diet. To find the optimal texture adjustment or diet for each person, it is always preferable to speak with a healthcare professional or speech-language therapist.

For seniors with particular nutritional needs, there are other dietary alterations besides textural changes that can be useful. Seniors with diabetes, for instance, may need to limit their intake of carbs or avoid meals with added sugars, while those with high blood pressure may need to watch their sodium intake. A certified dietician or healthcare professional can offer advice on how to adapt pureed foods to fit these particular dietary demands.

Overall, texture adjustments can be a useful tool for seniors and caregivers to make sure pureed foods are wholesome and safe. Caregivers can support their loved ones in maintaining their health and enjoying meals by taking into account each senior's specific dietary requirements and collaborating with healthcare professionals to design a meal plan.

Chapter 2: Tools And Equipment

- Pureeing Kitchen Essentials

There are a few kitchen necessities that might make the task of preparing meals for an elderly relative or friend easier and more effective. Here are some things to think about:

1. **Blender or food processor:**

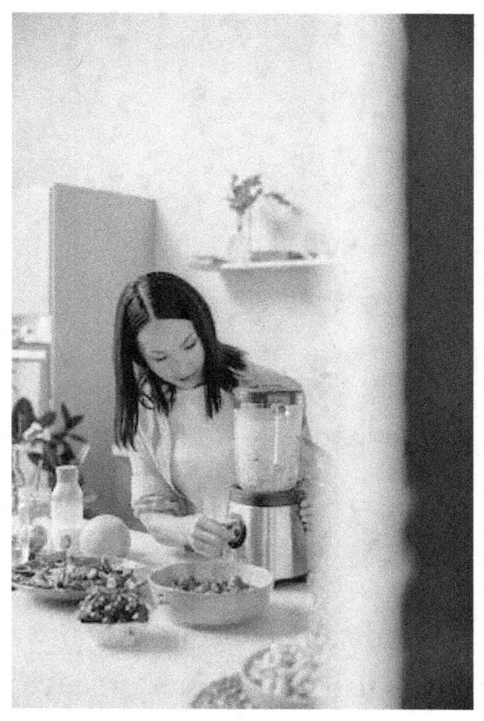

For pureeing food, a high-quality blender or food processor is required. To get the appropriate texture, look for a model with a strong motor and a variety of speed settings.

2. Strainer or Sieve:

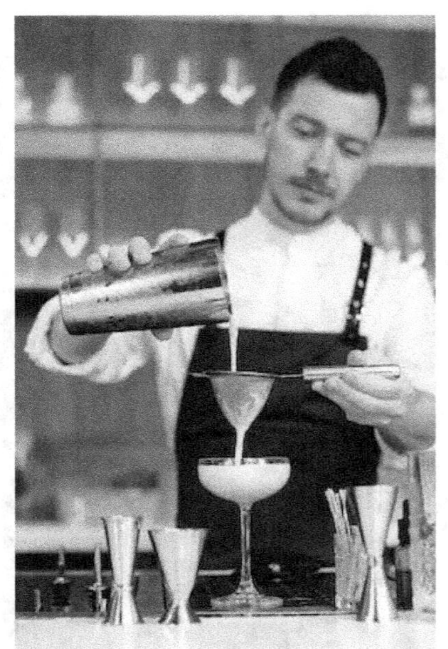

The pureed food can be cleaned of any undesired lumps or fibers using a strainer or sieve. Find a fine-mesh strainer or sieve that can capture even tiny food fragments.

3. *Measuring Cups and Spoons:*

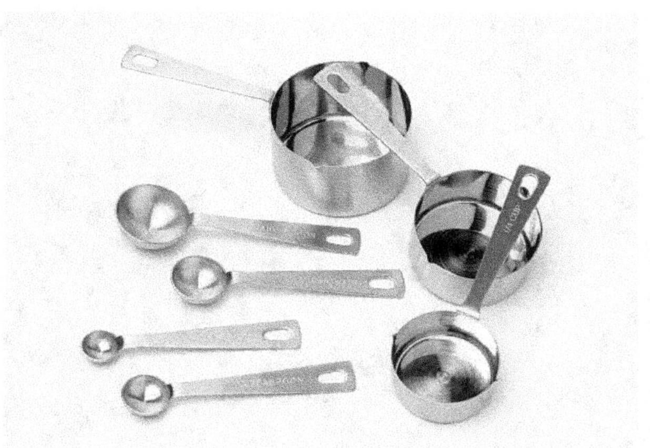

Preparing wholesome and well-balanced pureed meals requires precise measurement. To make sure you are using the right amount of ingredients, buy a set of measuring cups and spoons.

4. ***Cutting Board and Knife:***

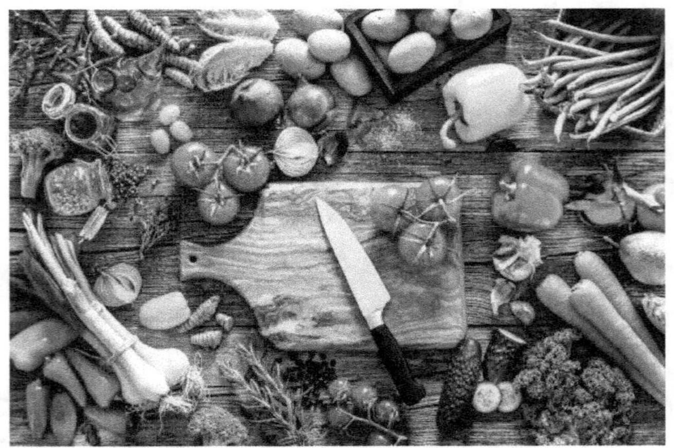

Before putting items in the blender or food processor, you may need to chop or dice them, even if you're pureeing food. This procedure can be made simpler and safer by using a cutting board and knife.

5. *Pots and Pans:*

To cook the ingredients before pureeing, you'll still need pots and pans. Look for non-stick cookware with handles that are comfortable to hold.

6. *Freezer Containers:*

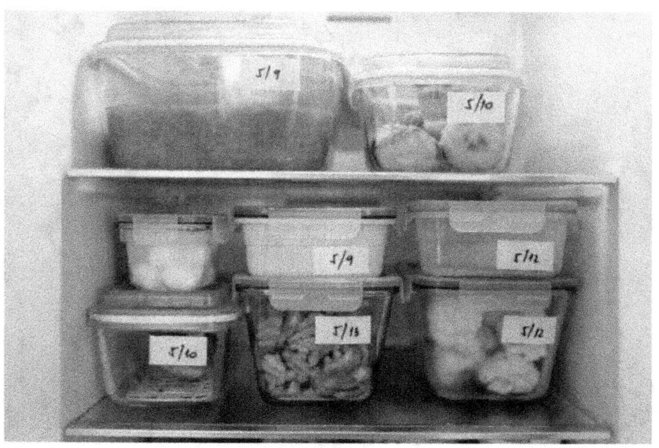

Buy freezer-safe containers to keep big amounts of pureed food in case you want to use them later. Look for storage-friendly, stackable containers that are simple to label.

Generally speaking, pureeing meals for elders may be done more quickly, safely, and effectively with the correct kitchen tools. Caregivers can make sure that the meals they are preparing for their loved ones are nourishing and well-balanced by spending money on high-quality supplies and instruments.

7. *Rubber Spatula:*

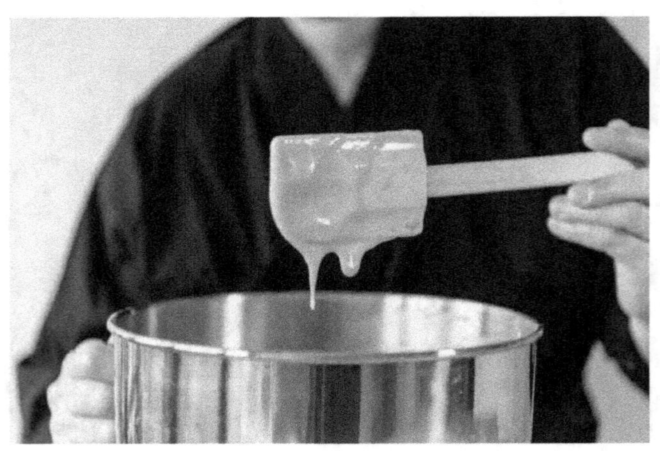

You can simply scrape food off the edges of the food processor or blender using a rubber spatula, ensuring that you receive all of the pureed food.

8. *Mixing Bowls:*

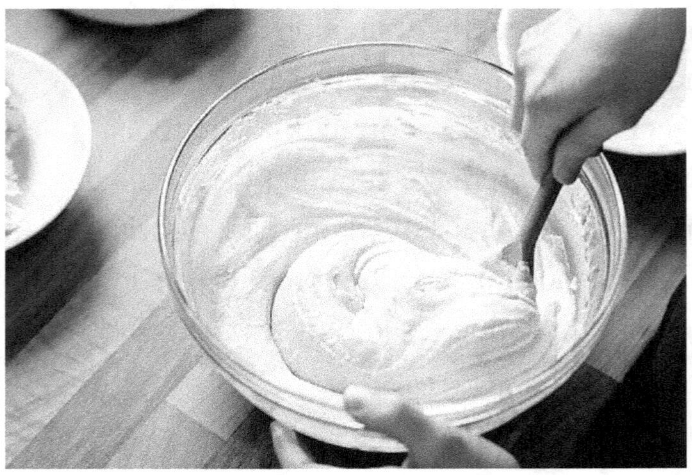

To combine ingredients or transfer pureed food
from the blender or food processor to a serving
plate, you may require mixing bowls.

9. *Immersion Blender:*

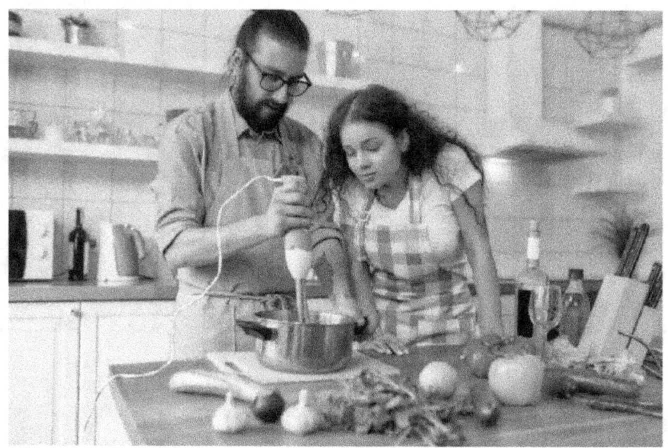

Instead of using a regular blender or food
processor, consider using an immersion blender.
It is a handheld blender that may be used to
purée tiny amounts of food right in the pot or
bowl.

10. *Electric Can Opener:*

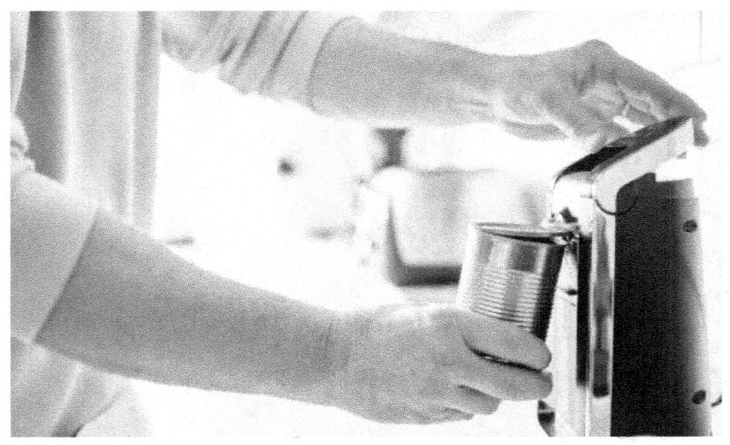

Seniors who have trouble using manual can openers may find an electric can opener to be a handy tool. It might make it simpler to open the cans of ingredients like fruit, beans, or vegetables.

11. *Food Mill:*

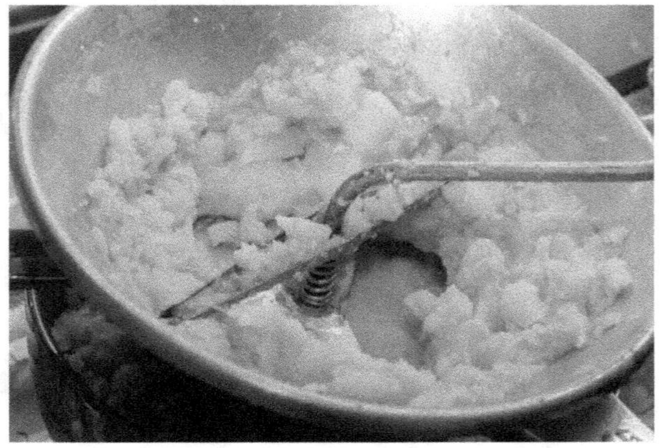

If you want a finer texture, a food mill is an additional alternative for pureeing food. A smoother puree will come from the removal of any seeds or skin from the meal.

12. *Food scale:*

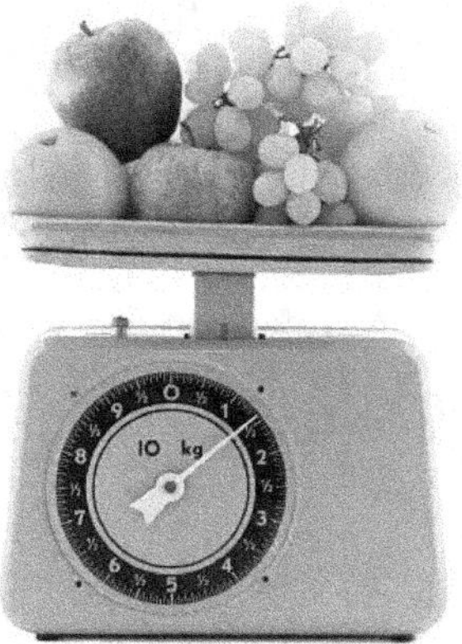

If you're preparing food according to a certain recipe or diet, a food scale can be beneficial for weighing out the ingredients.

Making wholesome and delectable pureed meals for seniors would be easier if you have these culinary necessities on hand. Never be hesitant to try out various flavors and textures to see what your loved one prefers. Additionally, as always, confirm that your meals are satisfying your loved one's dietary requirements by speaking with a medical professional or registered dietitian.

13. *Non-Slip Cutting Board:*
It's crucial to use a non-slip cutting board to avoid mishaps. As you chop or dice the ingredients, this will help keep the board in place.

14. *Silicone Ice Cube Trays:*

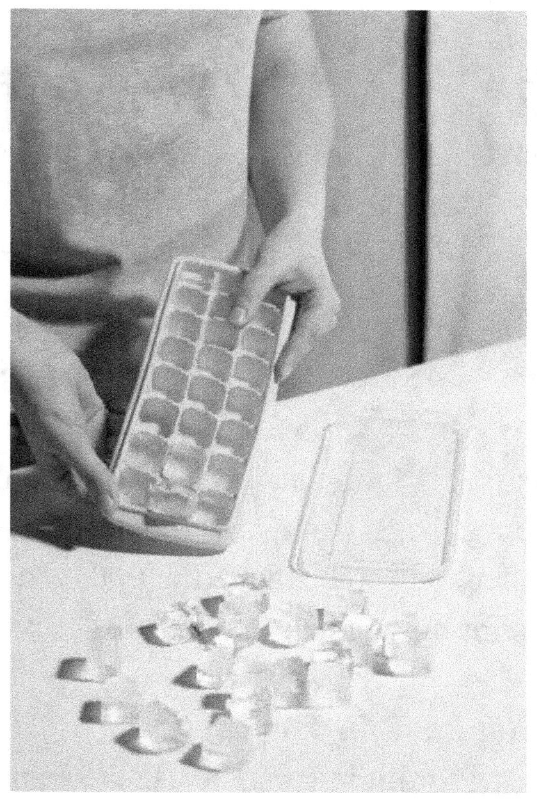

Silicone ice cube trays are a fantastic choice for portion-control freezing of pureed meals. The puree can be taken out of the tray once it has frozen and kept in a freezer-safe container.

15. *Food Storage Bags:*

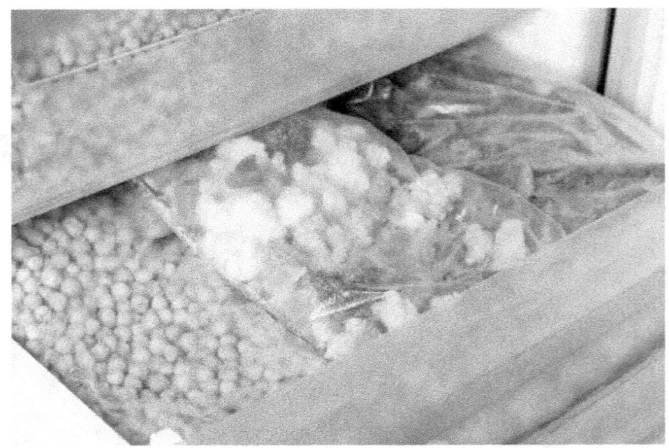

You can freeze food that has been pureed using food storage bags. Compared to containers, they are smaller and can be tagged with the date and contents for quick identification.

16. *Big Bowl for Mixing:*

A big bowl for mixing can be used to transfer pureed food to a container for storage.

17. *Colander:*

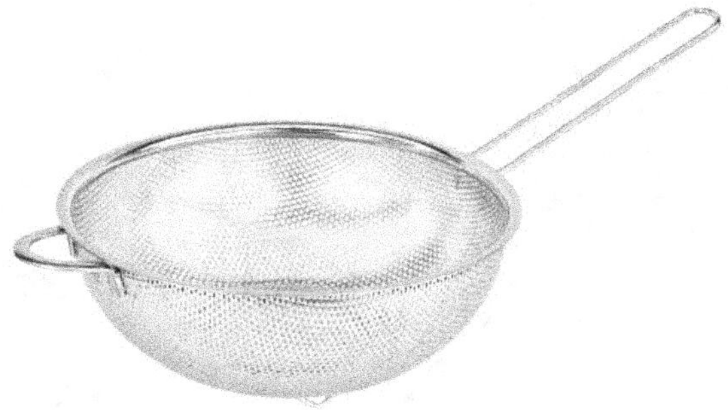

Before pureeing, cooked fruits or vegetables can be strained in a colander to eliminate extra liquid and produce a thicker puree.

18.***Whisk***:

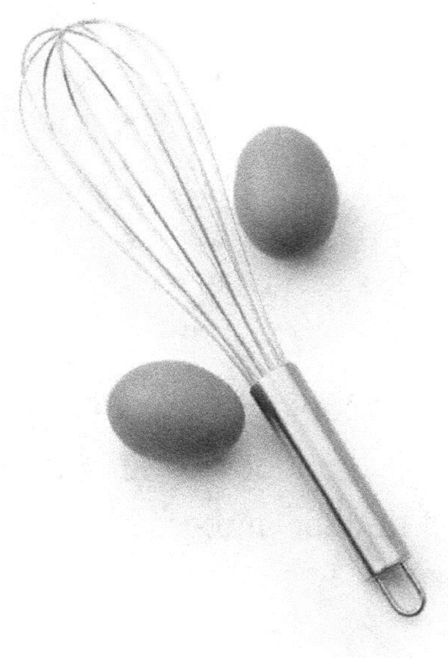

You can use a whisk to mix ingredients or to assist break up any lumps in a pureed dish.

19. *Garlic Press:*

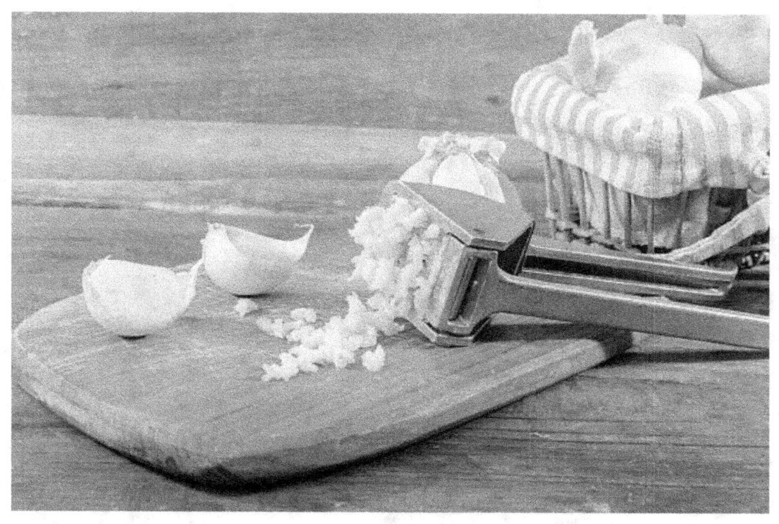

Using a garlic press to flavor pureed meals might be helpful. Without a knife, it may rapidly and efficiently crush garlic cloves.

20.*Oven Mitts:*

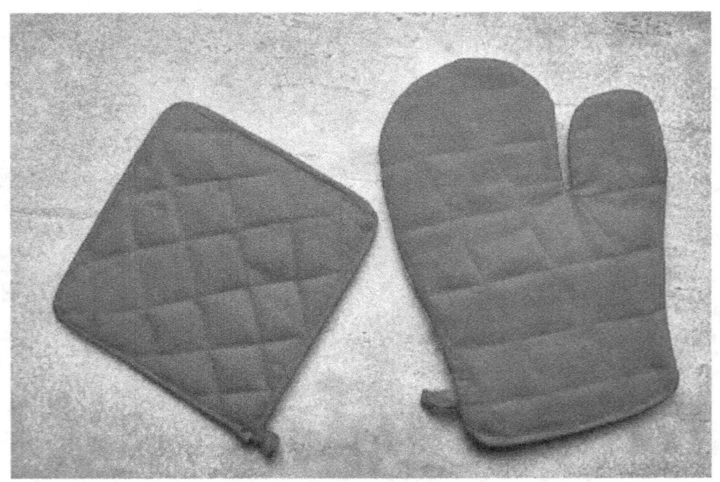

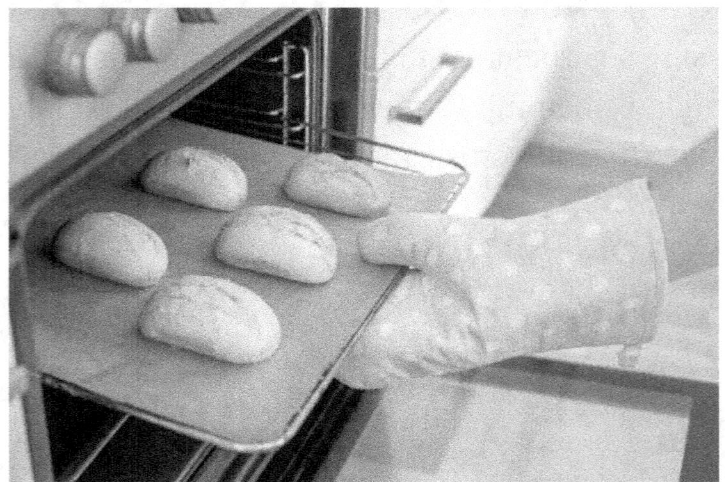

Having a pair of oven mitts on hand will help protect your hands from burns while cooking food in the oven.

These are merely a few illustrations of kitchen necessities that can facilitate and expedite the pureeing of food for senior citizens. You can make sure that you can feed your loved ones wholesome food by investing in these tools.

Meal trays with split parts might be useful when serving pureed meals to elderly people who have trouble feeding themselves. These can aid in separating various foods and avert spills.

21. *Blender bottles:*

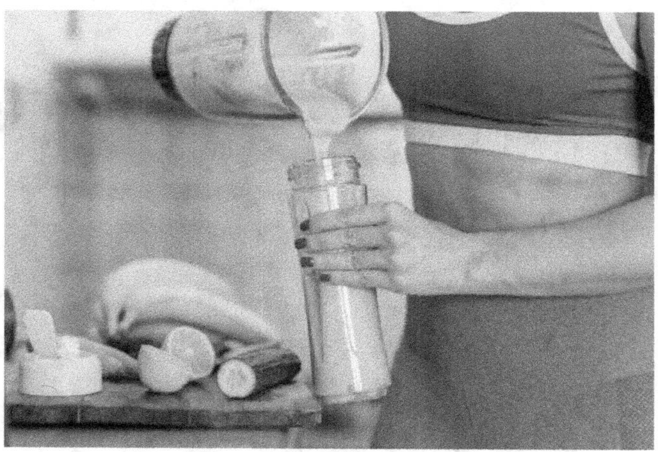

Blender bottles can be used to mix and store smoothies and other pureed liquids. They are portable. For seniors who are on the run or have trouble swallowing thick liquids, they can be a practical solution.

21. *Reusable Straws:*

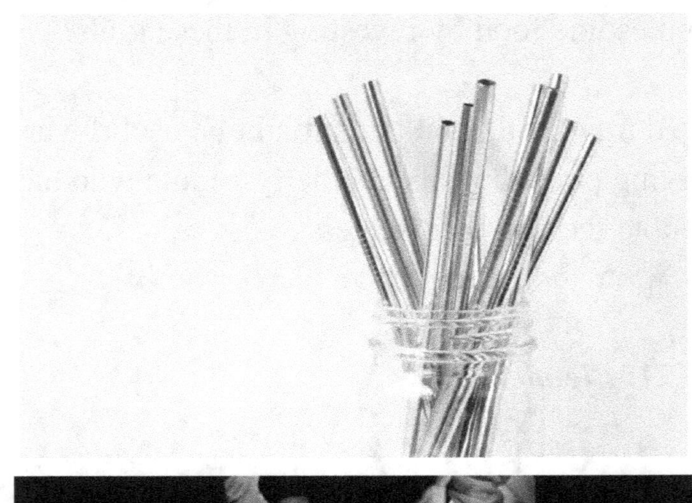

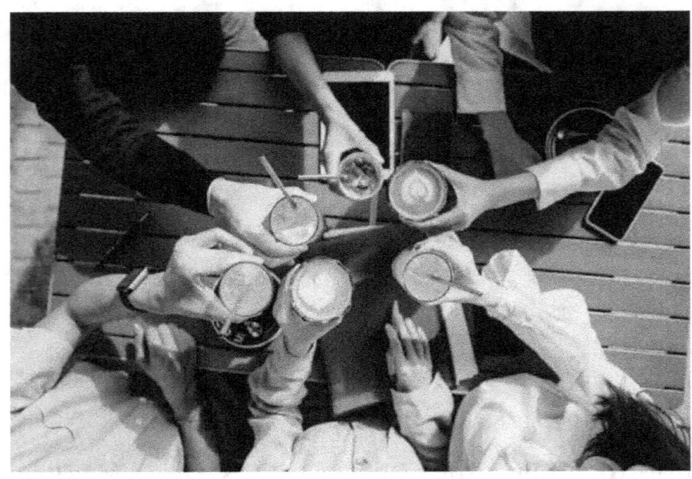

Due to their medical problems, some seniors may find it difficult to sip from normal straws. Wider-diameter reusable straws can make it simpler to consume thicker beverages.

22. *Jar openers:*

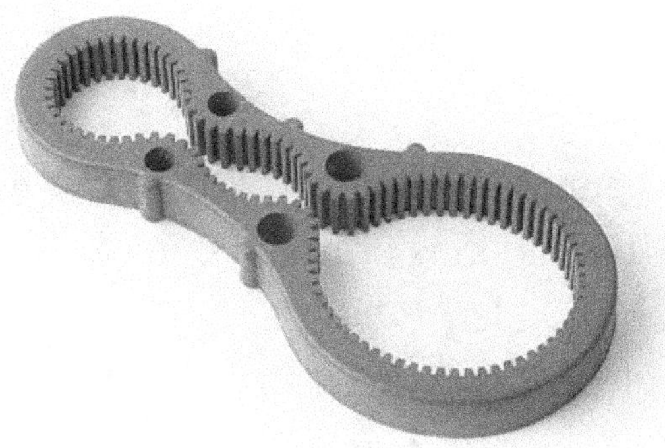

Seniors with arthritis or impaired grip strength may find it challenging to open jars. Jars of ingredients, such as sauces or spreads, can be opened more easily with jar openers.

23. *Vegetable Peeler:*

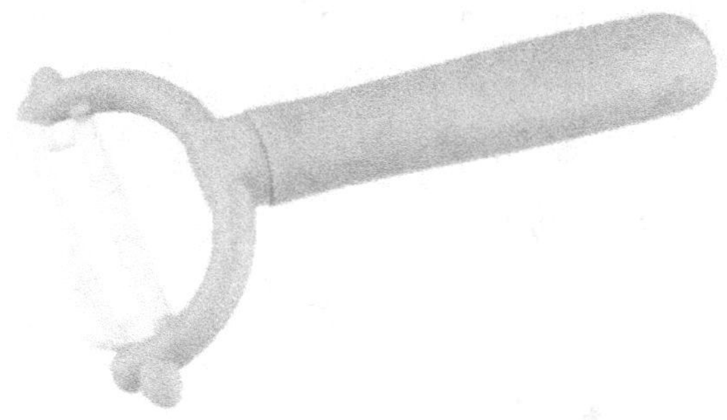

Before pureeing vegetables, it can be helpful to peel off their skins or tough outer layers with a vegetable peeler.

24.*Cheese grater:*

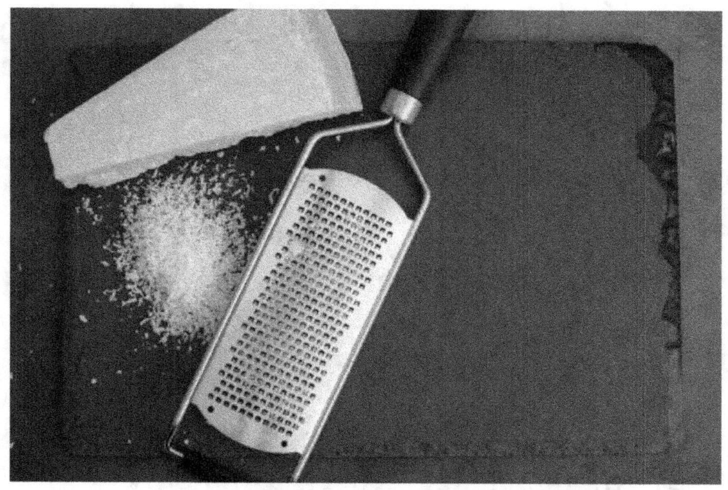

Before adding cheese to pureed foods, cheese can be grated into small pieces using a cheese grater.

25. ***Nutrient Additives:*** You can boost the nutritional value of pureed meals by including nutrient additives like protein powder or vitamin supplements.

You may further tailor pureed meals for seniors and make sure they are getting the nutrients they need by keeping these extra tools and ingredients on hand. Before incorporating any supplements

into meals, you should speak with a trained
nutritionist or healthcare professional.

26. A food processor is flexible equipment
that can be used to puree food, especially
in greater volumes. The components can
be swiftly chopped, blended, and pureed
to the required consistency.

27. An immersion blender, commonly
referred to as a hand blender, can be a
practical choice for pureeing smaller
quantities of food. It doesn't require
moving food to a blender because it can
be used right in the cooker or bowl.

28. *Chopper*:

Before adding herbs or nuts to pureed food, a
chopper might be handy for finely slicing the
items.

29. *Thermometer*:

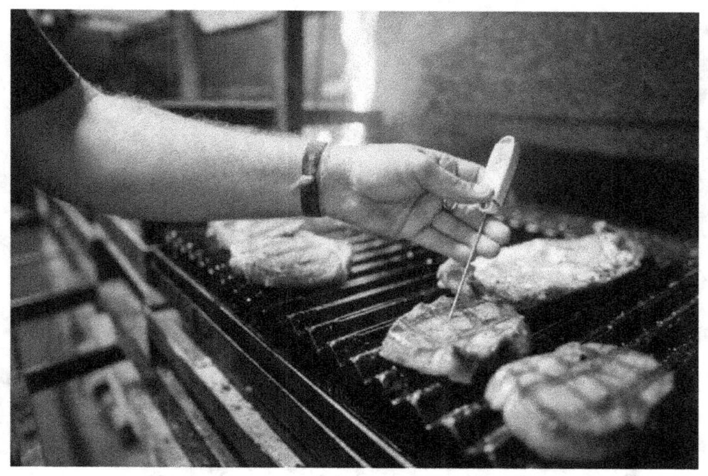

Using a thermometer will help you make sure that the meal is cooked to the right temperature.

30. *Storage Containers:*

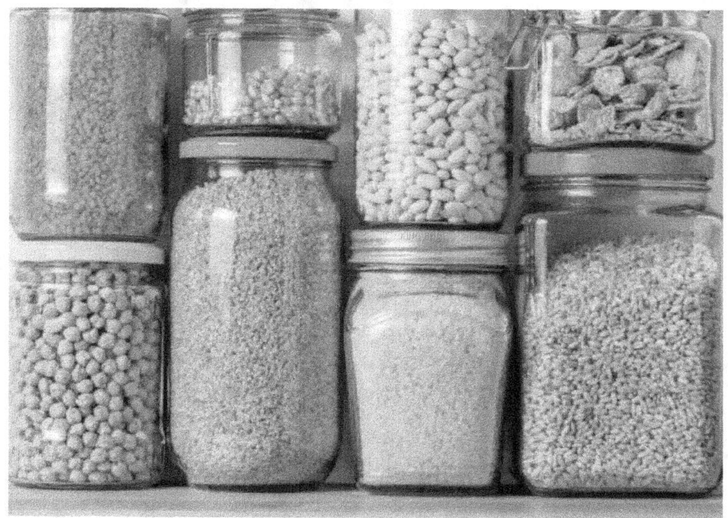

Pureed food can be kept in the freezer or refrigerator using storage containers. Pureed food can be frozen in glass jars or plastic containers that are marked as freezer-safe.

You may greatly simplify and speed up the process of pureeing food for elders by keeping these necessary items in your kitchen. It's crucial to spend money on durable kitchen equipment to guarantee the food you cook is both safe and of good quality.

31. ***Silicone molds:***

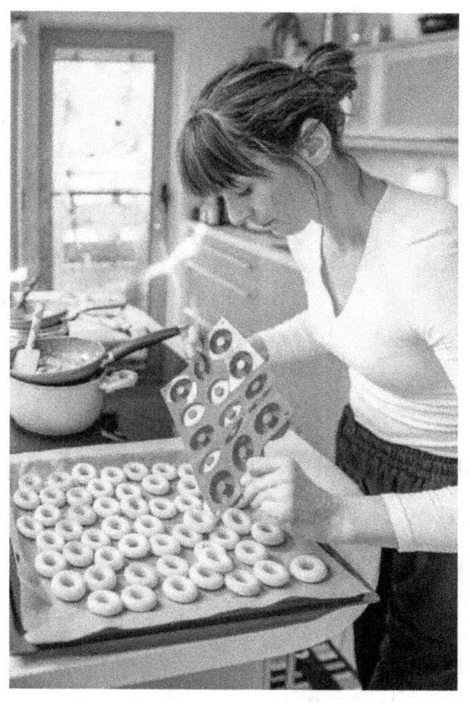

By using silicone molds to make uniform
servings of pureed food, it is easier to regulate
portion sizes and make sure that seniors are
eating the right amount of food.

32. *Electric pressure cooker:*

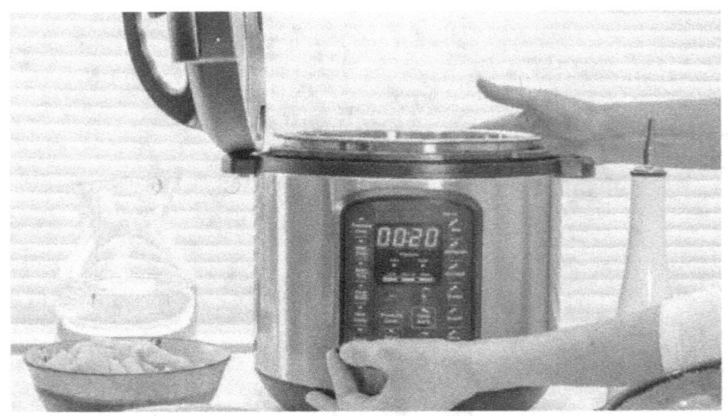

An electric pressure cooker is a useful piece of equipment for pre-pureeing cooking ingredients. It can shorten the cooking process and keep the food's nutrients intact.

33. *Steamer Basket:*

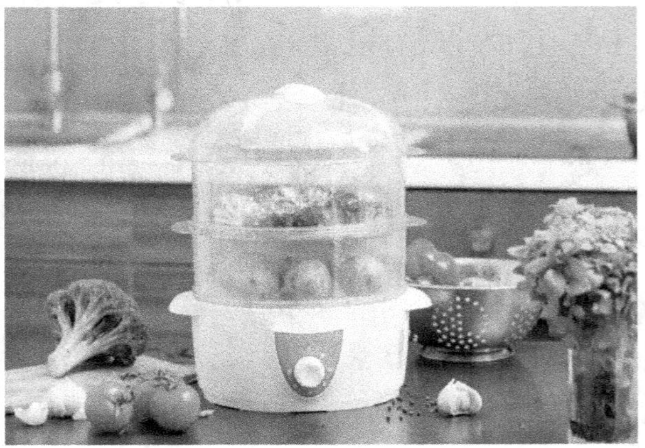

Vegetables can be steamed in a steamer basket before being pureed, helping to preserve their nutrients.

34. *Slow Cooker:*

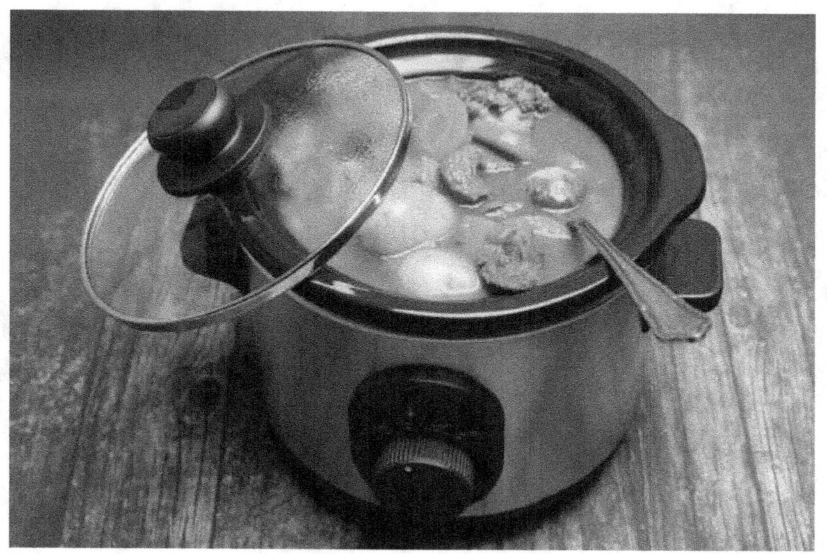

By cooking components for pureed meals over a longer period, a slow cooker produces meals that are tasty and tender.

You may make a greater range of pureed meals for seniors and tailor them to their dietary needs and tastes by using these extra kitchen items. Always make sure the equipment you use is secure and simple to use, especially for elderly people who might have trouble utilizing specific kitchen tools.

Furthermore, while the right equipment can make pureeing food simpler, it's equally crucial to make sure that the food is nutritionally sound and meets the dietary requirements of seniors. Preventing foodborne illness, entails utilizing a variety of fresh ingredients, adding various textures and flavors, and making sure the food is cooked to the proper temperature.

It's crucial to take into account any dietary restrictions or medical issues that can necessitate dietary changes when pureeing food for elders. For instance, senior citizens with diabetes may require low-sugar meals, while those with high blood pressure may need low-sodium meals.

Seniors should be included in the design of meals, and their tastes and cultural background should be taken into account. This can make sure they savor their meals and feel full afterward.

Overall, pureed food can be a significant component of a senior's diet and, with the right equipment and care, can be wholesome, delectable, and simple to prepare.

- Specialized Pureeing Equipment

Additionally, there are options for specialized equipment that can be especially useful for seniors with more complicated dietary needs when pureeing food. Here are a few instances:

Blender bottles are created to make mixing and blending ingredients simple. They can be used to make smooth, lump-free liquids, which can be useful for seniors who have dysphagia or difficulty swallowing.

1. Use a food mill to purée food into a smooth consistency. A food mill is a hand-cranked device. Seniors who enjoy their pureed meals with a slightly thicker consistency will find it especially useful.

2. Electric Food Mill: A motorized variant of a hand-cranked food mill, an electric food mill can be used to swiftly and easily purée food.

3. Baby food makers can be useful tools for rapidly and easily pureeing little volumes of food. They can quickly produce smooth purees and are made to be simple to operate.

4. Pre-packaged pureed meal kits that are specially made for elders are offered by several businesses. These kits often come with a selection of nutritiously sound and simple-to-prepare meals.

These solutions for specialist equipment can be beneficial for senior citizens who need more particular dietary changes or have trouble using conventional kitchen appliances. Before making any big dietary adjustments, it's crucial to conduct research, select equipment that is tailored to the user's needs, and speak with a healthcare provider.

Seniors who might have trouble cooking meals on their own have access to pre-made pureed food options in addition to specialized equipment. These alternatives can consist of pureed soups, fruits, vegetables, meats, and cereals.

It's crucial to choose pre-made pureed food options that are low in sodium and sugar and that offer a variety of nutrients. Additionally, it's crucial to make sure the food is safe to eat by checking the expiration dates.

However convenient pre-made pureed food options may be, they might not be as flavorful or wholesome as homemade pureed meals. Additionally, they might not satisfy the person's particular dietary requirements or preferences. The best method to choose the right diet for seniors is to speak with a certified dietitian and a member of the medical community.

Overall, the objective is to make sure that seniors are getting the right nutrition and enjoying their meals, whether you choose to prepare handmade pureed meals or choose pre-made options. Pureed food can be a valuable component of a senior's diet and can assist in preserving their health and well-being with the correct tools, equipment, and considerations.

Chapter 3: Preparing Pureed Food

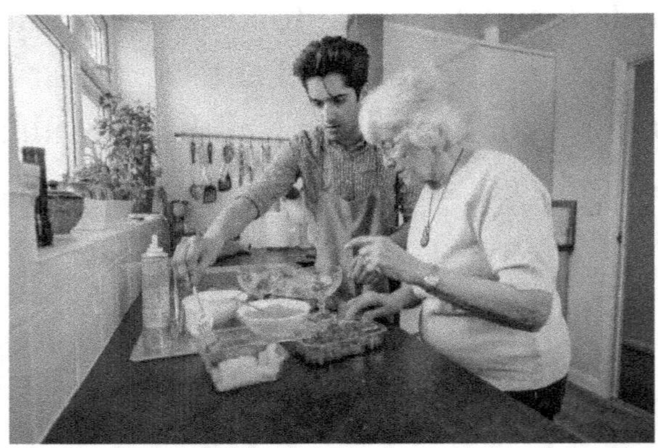

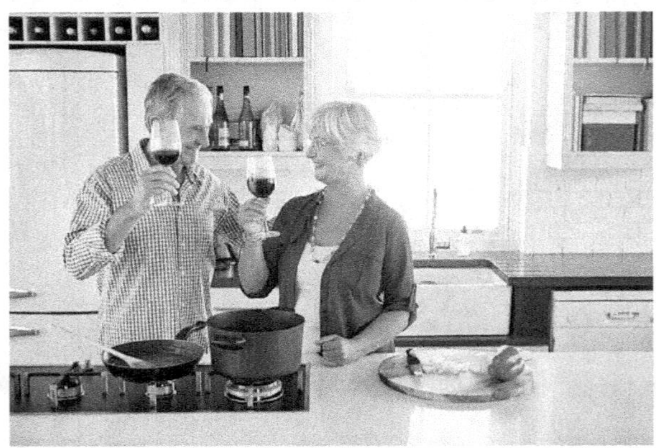

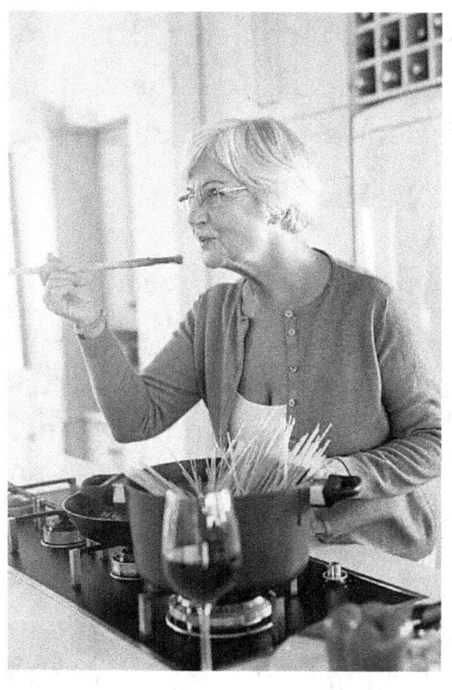

To guarantee that the texture and consistency of pureed food are appropriate for older citizens' needs, several additional considerations must be made when preparing it. Following are some suggestions for making pureed food:

1. Cut food into little pieces: To guarantee that food is pureed easily and uniformly, cut food into small, bite-sized pieces.

2. Cook food thoroughly: To make sure that the ingredients are soft and simple to puree, make sure that all of the ingredients are cooked completely.

3. Take out any bones, seeds, or skin before pureeing: To prevent any potential choking hazards, take out any bones, seeds, or skin from products including fruits, vegetables, and meats before pureeing.

4. Add liquids as necessary: You may need to add liquids like broth, milk, or water to get the correct consistency depending on the ingredients.

5. Use a food processor or blender: These appliances can swiftly and effectively combine ingredients to create a smooth puree, making them the greatest tools for pureeing meals.

6. If necessary, sift the pureed food to remove any pieces or fibers that might be challenging to swallow. This depends on the contents.

7. Chill food before serving: After food has been pureed, chillin it will help the meal solidify and attain a more appetizing texture.

These guidelines can help you make smooth, delectable pureed meals that are simple for elders to consume and process.

8. Label and date pureed food containers carefully to make sure they are used within the recommended time limit.

9. Portion and freeze: For greater convenience at mealtime, think about portioning pureed food into separate containers and freezing them for later use. Additionally, it can aid in reducing waste.

10. Reheat carefully: Pureed food should be reheated cautiously to avoid hot regions that could cause mouth burns. To make sure the meal is heated evenly all the way through, stir it frequently and use a thermometer.

11. Include nutrition boosters: To make sure elders are getting all the nutrients they require, think about including flaxseed, nutritional yeast, or protein powder in their pureed meals.

12. Add flavor and diversity: Use herbs, spices, and wholesome fats like avocado or olive oil to give pureed foods more taste and variation.

Consider food intolerances and allergies when creating pureed meals. If a senior has any food intolerances or allergies, make sure to avoid using those items.

13. Provide options: Even though some elders require pureed food, they should still have a say in what they eat. Provide a range of pureed options, and as much as possible, involve the senior in meal planning.

You may prepare pureed meals for seniors that are secure, nourishing, and pleasant while also catering to their dietary requirements and preferences by using these extra suggestions.

- Selection Of Fresh Ingredients

Making pureed meals for elders requires careful consideration of the freshness of the components. In addition to tasting better, fresh ingredients are more nutrient-dense than processed or canned foods. Following are some suggestions for choosing fresh ingredients:

- Opt for seasonal produce: Seasonal products are sometimes more inexpensive, fresher, and tastier than fruit that is not in season. It's a fantastic way to switch up your diet and explore different cuisines.

- Seek out vibrant hues: Colorful fruits and vegetables are frequently high in vitamins, minerals, and antioxidants. Choose food that is firm, ripe, and imperfect-free.

- Carefully study the labels of any prepackaged foods you buy to make sure they are low in sodium and sugar. Choose items that are manufactured with natural ingredients and entire foods.

- Purchase from local farmers: This is a terrific way to support your neighborhood and get fresh, in-season vegetables. Seniors may choose local vegetables because it is frequently grown without pesticides and other chemicals by local growers.

- Keep food safety in mind: To avoid contamination and spoiling, it's crucial to handle and store fresh products appropriately. Fruits and vegetables should be well washed before eating and should be kept in the refrigerator to preserve freshness.

You can make sure the pureed food you prepare for elders is both wholesome and delectable by using seasonal, fresh ingredients and practicing food safety.

Here are some extra pointers to bear in mind while selecting fresh ingredients for pureed meals in addition to the ones already mentioned:

- Select lean proteins for your pureed meals: Seniors may be more susceptible to heart disease and other health issues, so it's vital to select lean proteins like chicken, turkey, fish, and beans.

- Select healthy fats: For pureed meals, it's crucial to select healthy fats like olive oil, avocado, and almonds. Fats are a crucial component of a balanced diet.

- Choose low-glycemic carbohydrates: Carbohydrates provide you with energy, but you should choose low-glycemic varieties such as sweet potatoes, quinoa, and brown rice to help maintain stable blood sugar levels.

- Choose calcium-rich foods: Seniors may be in danger of osteoporosis when their bones deteriorate with age. To keep their bones strong, it's vital to choose calcium-rich foods like broccoli, kale, and yogurt.

- Take into account the person's nutritional requirements and preferences: Every senior is unique, therefore it's critical to consider their particular dietary requirements and preferences. You may need to modify their pureed meals if they have specific medical issues or allergies.

You may assist elders in maintaining their health and nutrition by choosing fresh, wholesome ingredients and tailoring pureed meals to match specific dietary needs.

Absolutely! You can maintain elders' health, stop malnutrition, and enhance their quality of life by making nourishing, individualized pureed meals

for them. Additional advice for preparing pureed
food for seniors is provided below:

- Refrain from using excessive amounts of
  salt: Seniors should consume less sodium
  because they may be at risk for high blood
  pressure. They should use herbs and
  spices to flavor their pureed food rather
  than too much salt.

Use healthy cooking techniques while preparing
the components for pureed meals, such as
steaming, boiling, or roasting. Steer clear of
deep-frying and excessive oil use.

- Be mindful of the texture: You might need
  to modify the texture of the person's
  pureed meals depending on their dietary
  requirements and preferences. To reach
  the appropriate consistency, combine or
  process the ingredients in a food
  processor. If necessary, add thickeners
  such as cornstarch or pureed beans.

Add variation to your pureed meals to keep seniors from getting bored and to make sure they're getting a variety of nutrients. To make their meals more enjoyable and nutrient-dense, try experimenting with various fruits, veggies, proteins, and whole grains.

- Speak with a certified dietitian: If you're unclear on how to prepare wholesome, nutrient-dense pureed meals for an elderly person, take their advice. They can offer advice on menu planning, dish creation, and making sure the senior's dietary requirements are met.

These guidelines will help you make scrumptious, nourishing pureed meals that promote senior citizens' health and wellbeing.

- Techniques for Preparing Pureed Foods

Various strategies might aid in producing a smooth and delectable texture while preparing pureed foods. Here are some tips for effective cooking:

- Roasting: Fruits and vegetables can have their natural sweetness and flavor enhanced by roasting them. Additionally, softening them can make pureeing easier.

- Boiling is a fantastic method for preparing components like potatoes, carrots, and other root vegetables so that they are soft and simple to puree.

- Steaming is a gentle cooking technique that can help ingredients maintain some of their nutrients and flavor. For meals that will be pureed, it's a terrific way to cook vegetables like broccoli, cauliflower, and carrots.

- Braise: Braise is a slow cooking method that results in a tasty purée and can be used to soften tough portions of meat.

- Simmering: Simmering is a mild cooking technique that can be used to soften and tenderize items like grains and lentils.

- Microwave: Using a microwave to heat tiny amounts of food for pureeing is a quick and simple method. For reheating frozen pureed meals, it is extremely helpful.

A delicate and tasty puree can be produced using the sous vide cooking technique, which includes cooking food in a temperature-controlled water bath.

You may prepare delicious and nourishing pureed meals for seniors that are simple to swallow and digest by employing these cooking methods.

- Adding Seasoning And Flavor

Although pureed food may be thought of as bland or unappetizing, seniors may find it to be more delicious with a little seasoning and flavoring. Here are some suggestions for seasoning and flavored food that has been pureed:

Use herbs and spices to enhance the flavor and scent of pureed foods. Think of incorporating spices like cinnamon, cumin, and paprika together with herbs like basil, parsley, and cilantro.

Adding healthy fats, such as coconut oil, avocado oil, or olive oil, can improve the flavor and texture of pureed meals.

Use low-sodium seasonings: Too much sodium can be hazardous to elders, so think about substituting Mrs. Dash, herbs, and spices with high-sodium seasonings.

- Include acid: A little vinegar or lemon juice can assist to enhance the flavors of pureed meals.

- Experiment with various ingredients: To give pureed meals variation, don't be scared to try various ingredients. To produce unique flavors and sensations, experiment with utilizing various veggies, fruits, and grains.

- Include sweetness: Seniors may have a sweet tooth, so try including sweetness in the form of honey, maple syrup, or fruit in pureed meals.

- Include umami: Umami, the fifth flavor, is sometimes characterized as savory. Mushrooms, soy sauce, or miso paste can all be used to improve the umami flavor of pureed foods.

You may prepare delectable, enticing pureed meals for seniors using these suggestions.

Chapter 4: Pureed Food Recipes

- Recipes for Breakfast

Here are a few simple-to-make, nutrient-dense recipes for pureed breakfast foods:

1. Pureed banana and oats

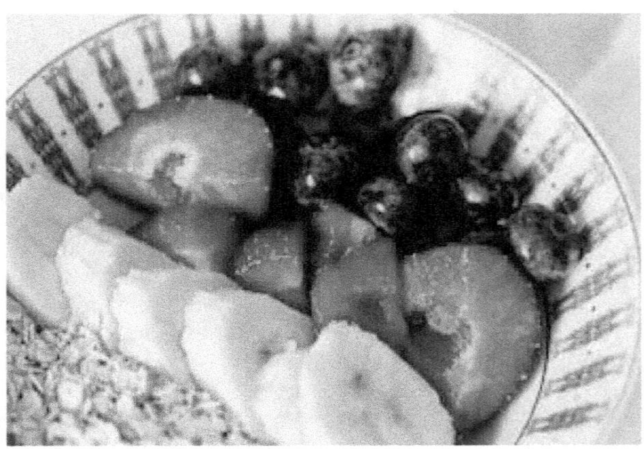

Ingredients:
- 1 ripe banana

-   1/4 cup milk or a milk substitute (such as almond milk) and 1/2 cup cooked oatmeal.
-   To taste cinnamon

Instructions:

- Place all ingredients in a blender or food processor and pulse until completely smooth.
- Present hot.

2. *Pureed scrambled eggs and cheese*

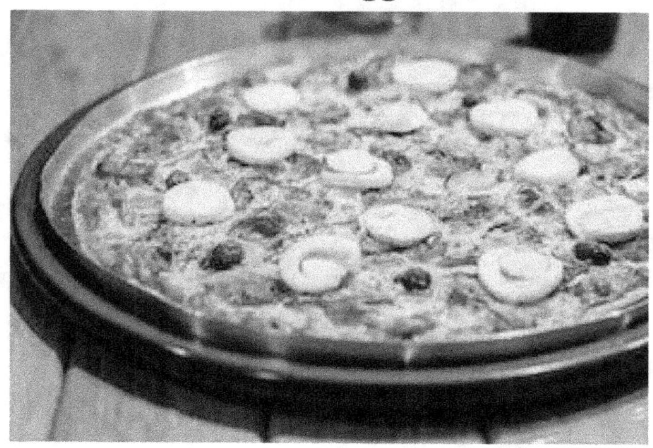

Ingredients:

-   two eggs.
-    One-fourth cup of milk or a milk substitute (such as soy milk)

- 1/4 cup of cheese, shredded
- To taste, salt and pepper

Instructions:
- Crack the eggs into a bowl, then whisk in the milk, salt, and pepper.
- Add the egg mixture to a nonstick pan that is already heated over medium heat.
- Add the shredded cheese after the eggs are cooked until they are set.
- After the cheese has melted, transfer the mixture to a food processor or blender.
- Blend till fluid.
- Present hot.

3. ***Pureed Apple Cinnamon***

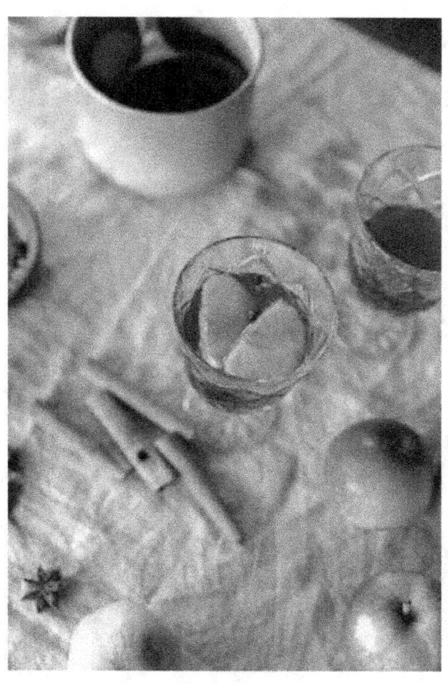

- 1 diced and peeled apple, along with 1/4 cup water.
- To taste cinnamon

Instructions:

- Fill a small pot with apples and water, and then bring to a boil.
- Lower the heat to a low setting and cook the apple for several minutes.
- Taste-testing add cinnamon.

- Transfer the mixture to a blender or food processor, and then pulse it until it is smooth.
- Present hot.

These pureed breakfast recipes are easy to make, filling, and adaptable to diverse tastes and dietary requirements.

4. Pureed sweet potatoes

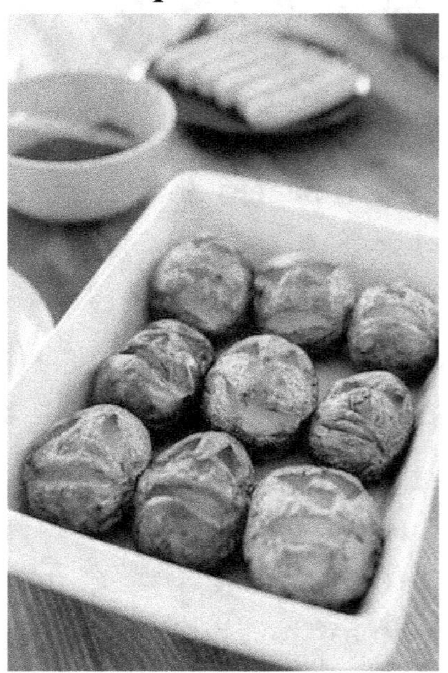

Ingredients:

- 1 sweet potato, diced, with the skin removed; 1/2 cup milk or milk substitute (such as coconut milk);
- 1/2 teaspoon of cinnamon
- 1 tbsp honey - 1/2 tsp ginger

Instructions:
To make sweet potatoes soft, steam or boil them.
- Combine the sweet potato, milk, cinnamon, ginger, and honey in a food processor or blender.
- Blend till fluid.
- Present hot.

5. Pureed Blueberry Yogurt

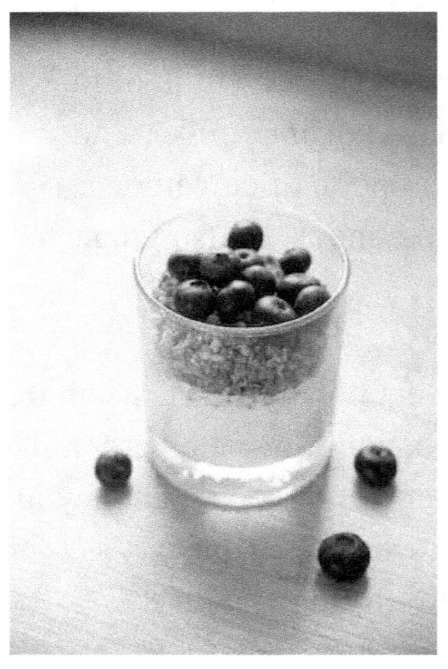

Ingredients:

- half a cup of blueberries
- 1/2 cup Greek yogurt, plain
- One-fourth cup of milk or a milk substitute (such as soy milk)
- 1 teaspoon honey

Instructions:

- In a blender or food processor, combine blueberries, Greek yogurt, milk, and honey.

- Purée until fluid.
- Present cold.

These nutrient-dense and simple-to-prepare pureed breakfast recipes are ideal for seniors who might have trouble chewing or swallowing solid foods.

6. *Fruit Puree And Cottage Cheese*

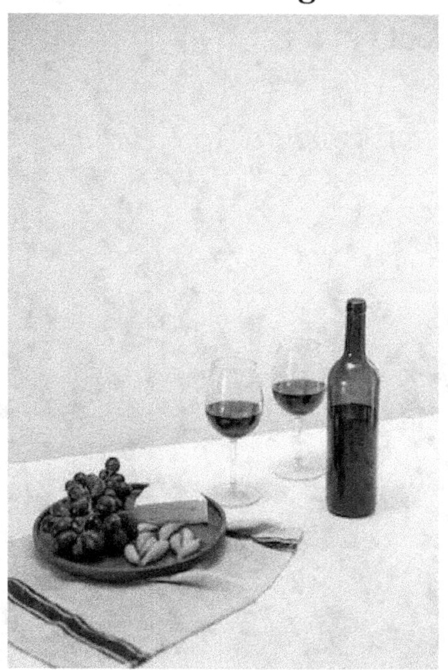

Ingredients:
- half a cup of cottage cheese.

- 1/2 cup chopped fresh fruit, such as bananas, strawberries, or peaches
- 1 tablespoon honey

Instructions:

- Cottage cheese, fruit, and honey should all be combined in a food processor or blender.
- Purée until fluid.
- Present cold.

7. *Pureed Avocado And Tomato*

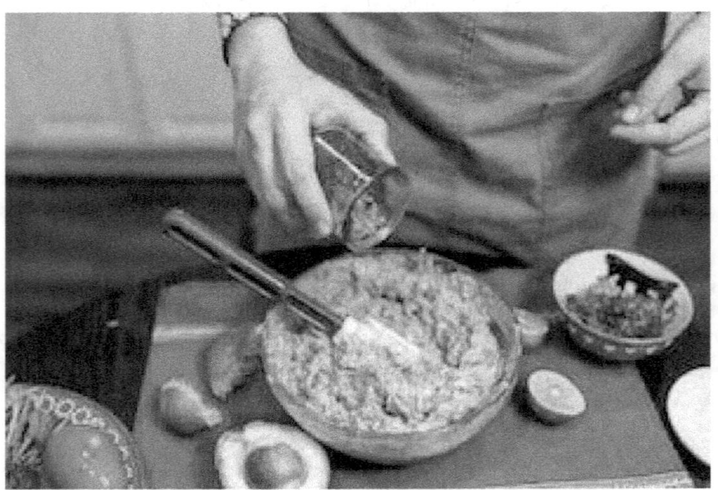

Ingredients:

- A single, ripe avocado

- 1/2 cup tomatoes, diced
- Salt and pepper to taste with 1/4 cup of
  water

Instructions:
- Halve the avocado, then remove the pit.
- Place the avocado flesh in a food
  processor or blender.
- Include water, salt, pepper, and diced
  tomatoes.
- Blend till fluid.
- Present cold.

These nutrient-dense pureed breakfast recipes
are ideal for seniors who might have trouble
chewing or swallowing solid foods because they
are simple to ingest. Additionally, they are easily
adaptable to diverse dietary requirements and
tastes.

-   Recipes For Lunch and Dinner

Dinner/Lunch Recipes:

1. ***Pureed Chicken And Vegetables***

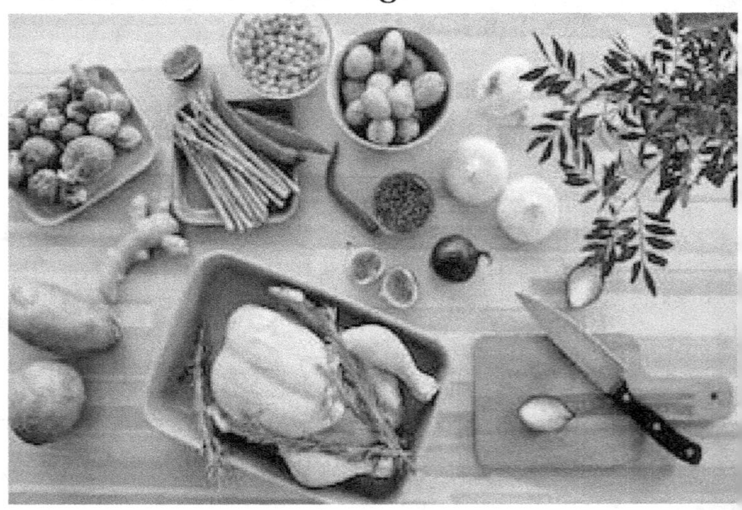

Ingredients:

-   Half a cup of chopped, cooked chicken
-   1/2 cup of mixed, cooked veggies, such as carrots, peas, and green beans

-   1/4 cup of vegetable or chicken broth, plus
    salt & pepper to taste

Instructions:

-   • In a blender or food processor, combine
    the chicken, veggies, broth, salt, and
    pepper.
-   • Purée until fluid.
-   • Present hot.

2. *Pureed Lentil And Sweet Potato*

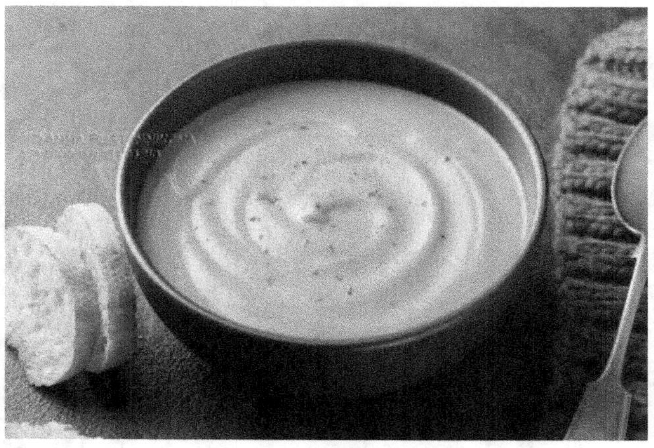

Ingredients:

-   1/2 cup mashed cooked sweet potato and
    1/2 cup cooked lentils

- 1/4 cup vegetable broth, 1/4 teaspoon each of cumin and coriander
- To taste, salt and pepper

Instructions:

- In a blender or food processor, combine the lentils, sweet potato, broth, cumin, coriander, salt, and pepper.
- Purée until fluid.
- Present hot.

3. *Pureed Beef With Potatoes*

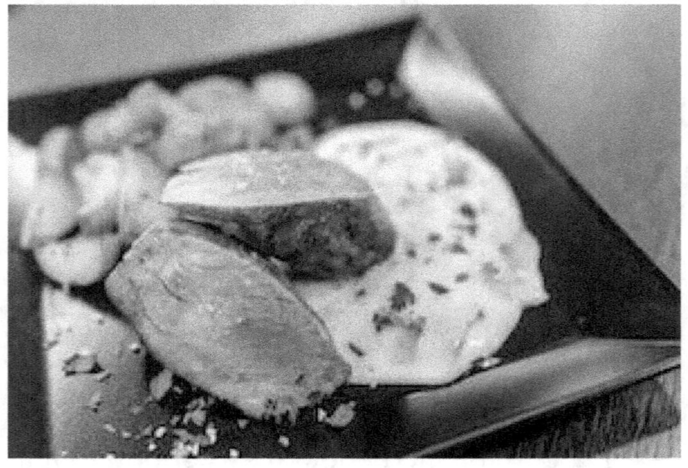

Ingredients:

- 1/4 cup beef or veggie broth, salt, and pepper to taste.

-   1/2 cup cooked ground beef.
-   1/2 cup cooked mashed potatoes.

Instructions:
- In a blender or food processor, combine the ground beef, mashed potatoes, stock, salt, and pepper.
- Purée until fluid.
- Present hot.

These pureed meal recipes for lunch and dinner are simple to prepare, and they can be made ahead of time and frozen or refrigerated for later use. Additionally, they are easily adaptable to diverse dietary requirements and tastes.

Here are some additional recipes for pureed lunch and dinner foods:

4. Soup With Carrots And Ginger

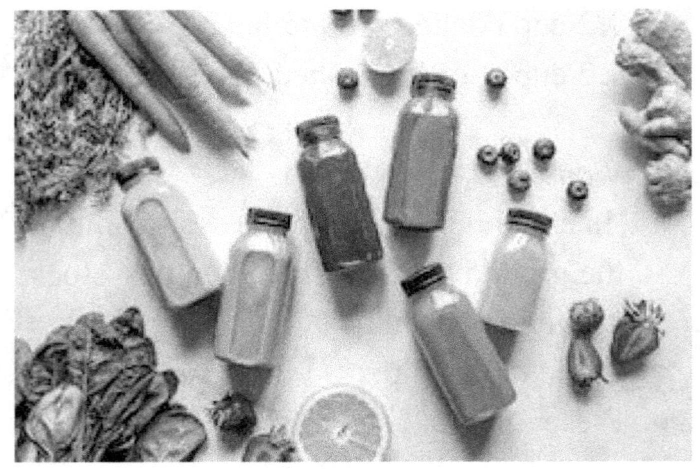

Ingredients:

- 1 lb. peeled and sliced carrots;
- 1 tbsp. grated fresh ginger;
- 2 cups chicken or veggie broth; and
- 1/2 cup heavy cream.
- To taste, salt and pepper

Instructions:

- Combine the carrots, ginger, and broth in a big pot. Bring to a boil, then lower the heat and simmer the carrots for 20 to 25 minutes, depending on their tenderness.

- After letting the mixture cool a bit, puree it in a blender or food processor until it's smooth.

- Add cream to the saucepan with the mixture that has been pureed, then season with salt and pepper to taste.

- Serve the soup after reheating it gently.

5. *Puree Salmon And Sweet Potatoes*

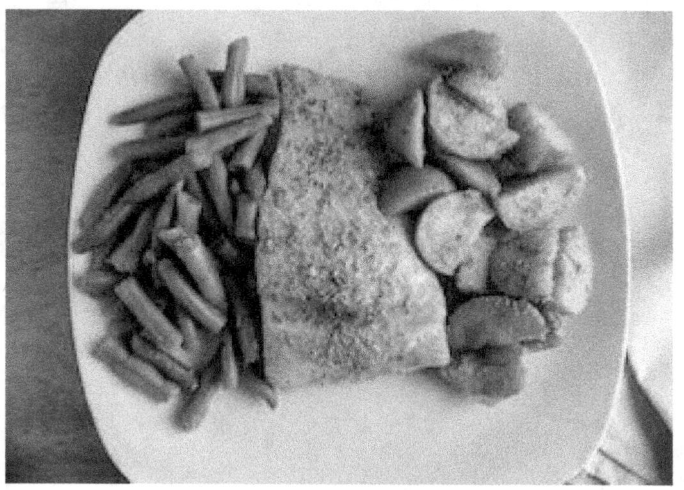

Ingredients:

- Half a pound of cooked salmon
- 1/2 cup mashed, cooked sweet potatoes

- 1/4 cup of vegetable or chicken broth
- 1/4 teaspoon of garlic powder
- To taste, salt and pepper

Instructions:
- Combine cooked salmon, mashed sweet potatoes, broth, garlic powder, salt, and pepper in a blender or food processor.
- Purée until fluid.
- Warm up the mixture by reheating it over low heat.

6. *Puree vegetables And beans*

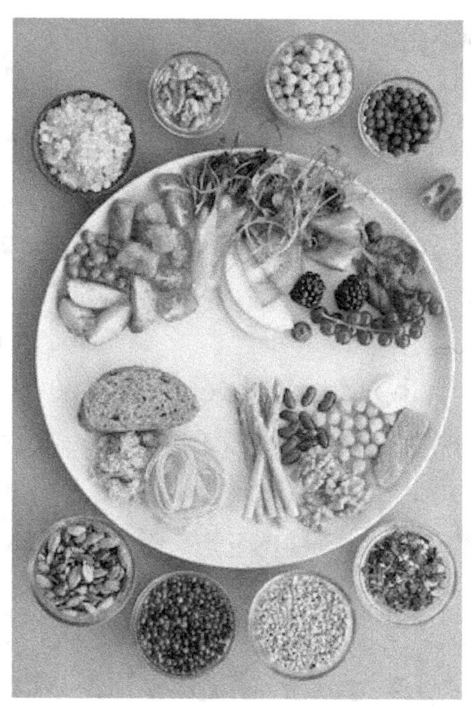

Ingredients:

- 1 can of rinsed and drained mixed beans;
- 1 cup of chopped mixed veggies, including celery, carrots, and zucchini.
- 1/4 cup of vegetable or chicken broth, plus salt & pepper to taste

Instructions:

- Combine mixed beans, mixed veggies, broth, salt, and pepper in a blender or food processor.
- Purée until fluid.
- Warm up the mixture by reheating it over low heat.

Seniors who have trouble chewing or swallowing solid foods might enjoy these flavorful and nutrient-rich lunches and dinner pureed food dishes. They are also fantastic for people on a diet of soft or pureed foods.

7. Creamy Mushroom Puree

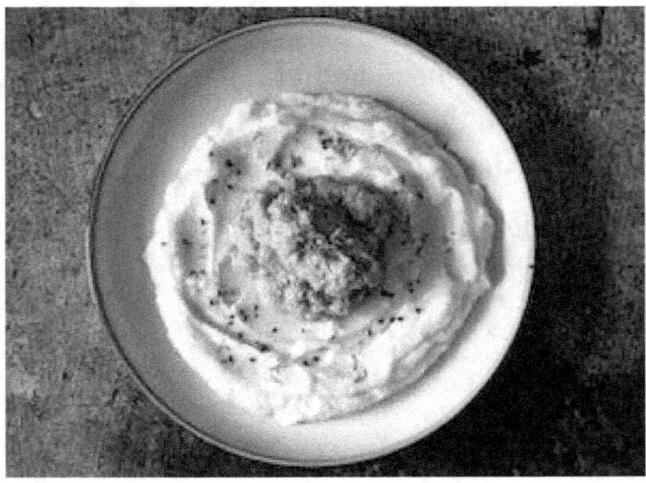

Ingredients:

- 1 pound chopped mushrooms; 1/2 cup heavy cream.
- 2 tablespoons of unsalted butter
- 1/4 cup of chicken or veggie broth
- 1/8 teaspoon dried thyme
- To taste, salt and pepper

Instructions:

- To begin, melt butter in a big pan over medium heat. Add the chopped mushrooms and simmer for a further 5-7 minutes, or until they are soft and have released their moisture.

- Add the broth, either chicken or vegetable, and simmer for an additional 2-3 minutes.

- After allowing the liquid to gradually cool, puree it in a blender or food processor until it's completely smooth.

- Add heavy cream, dried thyme, salt, and pepper to the pureed mixture before adding it back to the pan and heating on low until heated through.

- Present hot.

8. *Pureed Lentil And Carrot*

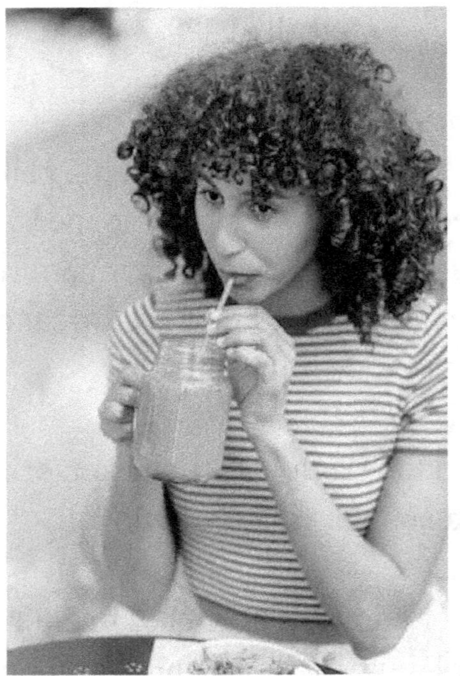

Ingredients:

- 1 cup washed and drained red lentils;
- 2 cups water or vegetable broth;
- 2 big carrots;

- 1/2 chopped onion; and
- 2 minced garlic cloves.
- 2 tablespoons olive oil
- A half teaspoon of ground cumin
- A dash of salt and pepper

Instructions:

- Heat the olive oil in a big pot over medium heat. Sauté the onion and garlic for two to three minutes, or until tender.

- Stir in the cumin and continue to sauté for an additional 2-3 minutes.

- Fill the saucepan with rinsed lentils, water, or vegetable broth, and bring to a boil.

- Lower the heat to low and simmer the mixture for 20 to 25 minutes, or until the carrots and lentils are tender.

- After allowing the mixture to cool slightly, smooth it out in a blender or food processor.

- Add salt and pepper to the pureed mixture before adding it back to the pot and heating on low until heated all the way through.

- Present hot.

These pureed meal dishes for lunch and dinner are simple to prepare and keep for a few days in the refrigerator. They are an excellent method to give seniors the nourishment they require while still allowing them to enjoy scrumptious and savory meals.

9. Pureed Chicken With Sweet Potato

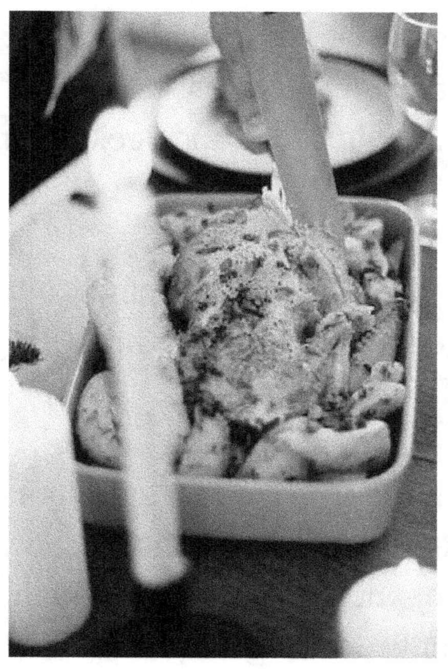

- 2 skinless, boneless chicken breasts
- 2 big, peeled, and sliced sweet potatoes
- 2 cups chicken or veggie broth
- 1/4 cup heavy cream
- 1/4 tsp ground cinnamon
- 2 tablespoons unsalted butter
- To taste, salt and pepper

Instructions:

- Heat the butter in a large pot over medium heat. Sweet potatoes should start to soften after being added and cooked for 5-7 minutes after that.

- Fill the saucepan with chicken breasts and vegetable or chicken broth. Bring to a boil.

- Lower the heat to low and simmer the mixture for 15 to 20 minutes, or until the sweet potatoes are tender and the chicken is cooked through.

- Take out the chicken breasts and set them aside.

- Blend the sweet potato mixture in a blender or food processor until it is completely smooth after allowing it to cool somewhat.

- Add heavy cream, cinnamon powder, salt, and pepper to the pot with the mixture that has been pureed. Heat on low until well warmed.

- Combine the cooked chicken breasts in the sweet potato purée after shredding.

- Present hot.

10.*Pureed Beef With Carrots*

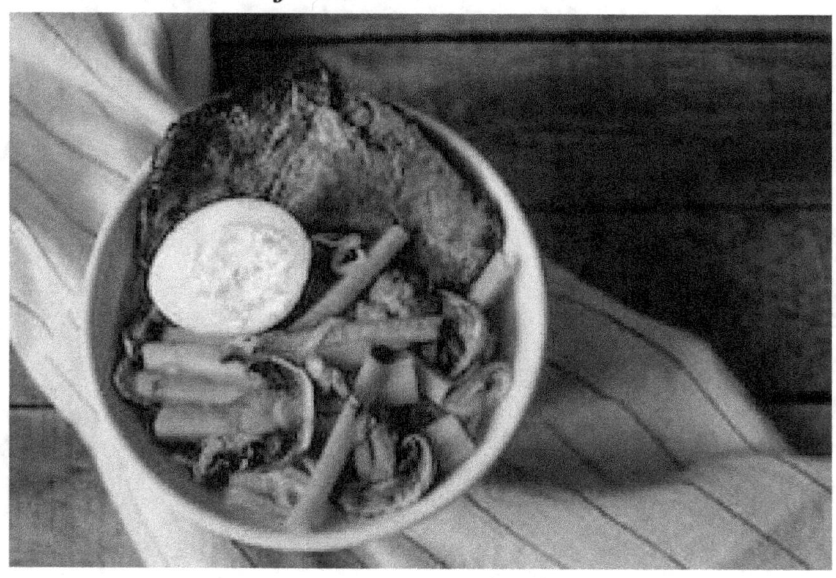

Ingredients:

- 1 pound of ground beef;
- 2 big carrots;
- 1/2 chopped onion.

- 2 minced garlic cloves
- 2 cups of vegetable or beef broth
- 2 tablespoons of olive oil
- To taste, salt and pepper

Instructions:

- Heat the olive oil in a big pot over medium heat. Sauté the onion and garlic for two to three minutes, or until tender.

- Stir in the chopped carrots and cook for a further 2-3 minutes.

- Stir in the ground meat and heat it until it is browned.

- Add the broth, either beef or vegetable and bring to a boil.

- Lower the heat and simmer the mixture for 15 to 20 minutes, or until the meat is thoroughly cooked and the carrots are tender.

- After allowing the mixture to cool slightly, smooth it out in a blender or food processor.

- Add salt and pepper to the pureed mixture before adding it back to the pot and heating on low until well heated.

- Present hot.

This nutrient- and protein-rich pureed meal dishes for lunch and dinner are ideal for seniors who require a soft diet. By altering the type of meat or broth used, they can simply be changed to accommodate various dietary requirements.

11. Recipe For Creamy Chicken And Vegetable Puree

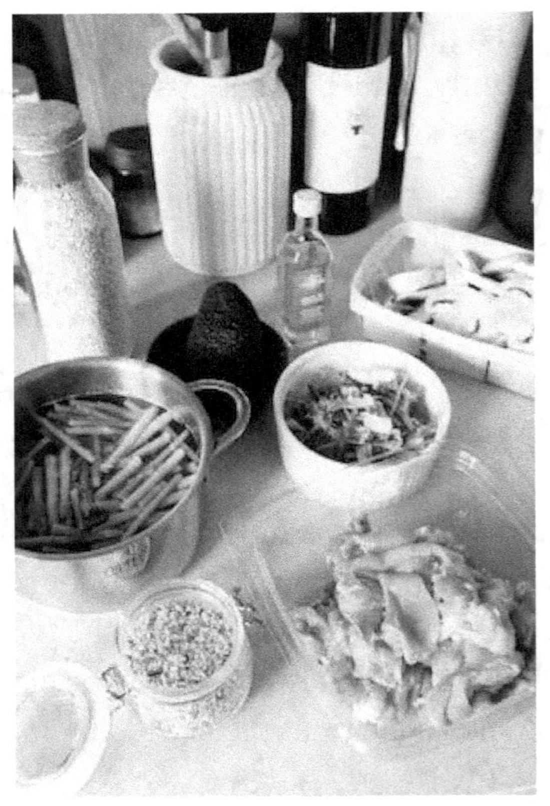

Ingredients:
- 2 cups of mixed veggies (carrots, green beans, peas),
- 1 cup of milk,
- 1 pound of boneless, skinless chicken breast, cubed
- Butter, 2 tablespoons
- 2 tbsp. all-purpose flour

- To taste, salt and pepper

Instructions:

- Combine the chicken, mixed veggies, and chicken broth in a big pot. After bringing it to a boil, lower the heat to a simmer.

- Cook for 20 to 25 minutes, or until the veggies are soft and the chicken is thoroughly cooked.

- Remove from heat and let it briefly cool.

- Puree the chicken and veggies in a blender or food processor until they are completely smooth.

- Melt the butter in a saucepan over medium heat.

- Cook for 1-2 minutes after adding the flour and stirring to incorporate.

- Add the milk little by little while continuing to stir until the mixture thickens.

- Stir together the pureed chicken and veggies in the pot.

- To taste, add salt and pepper to the dish.

- Present hot.

Note: You can change the flavor of this recipe to your liking by substituting other veggies or by adding herbs and spices.

12. Recipe For Butternut Squash And Carrot Puree

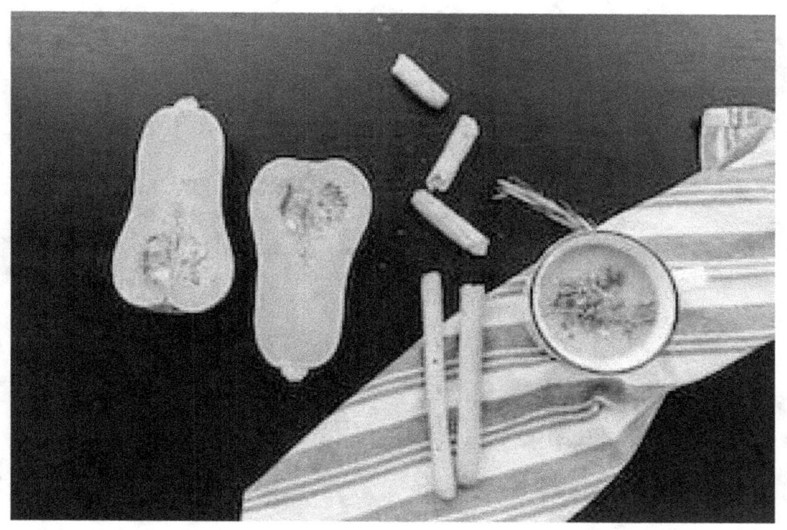

Ingredients:

- 1 diced butternut squash,
- 3 sliced carrots,
- 2 cups low-sodium vegetable broth, and -
- 1/4 cup heavy cream.
- butter, 2 tablespoons
- To taste, salt and pepper
- Combine the butternut squash, carrots, and vegetable broth in a big pot. After bringing it to a boil, lower the heat to a simmer.

Instructions:

- Cook the vegetables for 20 to 25 minutes, or until they are soft.

- Remove from heat and let it briefly cool.

- Puree the veggies in a blender or food processor until they are smooth.

- Melt the butter in a saucepan over medium heat.

- Include the pureed vegetables and blend by stirring.

- Stir continuously while gradually adding the heavy cream until thoroughly cooked.

- To taste, add salt and pepper to the dish.

- Present hot.

Note: You can alter this recipe by using various kinds of squash or by enhancing the flavor with spices like cinnamon or nutmeg.

- Recipes For Snacks And Desserts

1. *Recipe For Mango And Avocado Puree*

Ingredients:
- 1/4 cup plain Greek yogurt,
- 1 ripe mango, chopped and peeled;
- 1 ripe avocado, peeled and pitted.
- 1 teaspoon of honey

Instructions:
- Blend or pulse the mango and avocado until completely smooth.

- Blend in the honey and Greek yogurt until thoroughly mixed.

- Serve chilled as a light dessert or snack.

Note: To change this dish and add some zing to the flavor, add a squeeze of lime juice or a dash of chile powder.

2. *Recipe For Creamy Berry Puree*

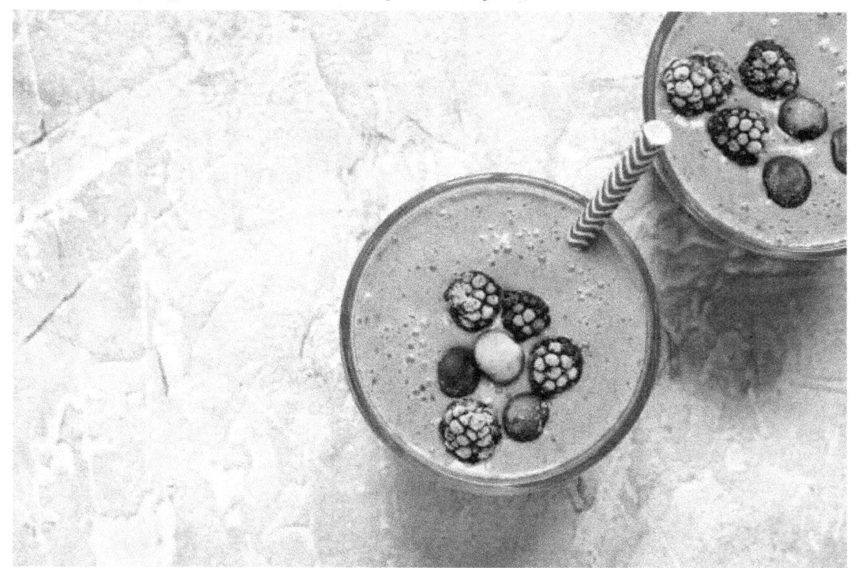

Ingredients:

-   1/4 cup plain Greek yogurt,
-   1 ripe banana,
-   1 cup mixed berries (strawberries, raspberries, and blackberries), and
-   1 cup mixed berries.
-   1 teaspoon of honey

Instructions:

- Puree the banana and mixed berries in a blender or food processor until they are completely smooth.

- Blend in the honey and Greek yogurt until thoroughly mixed.

- Serve chilled as a dessert or a nutritious snack.

Note: You can alter this recipe by switching up the berries or by adding a little almond milk for a creamier texture.

3. *Recipe For Avocado And Tomato Puree*

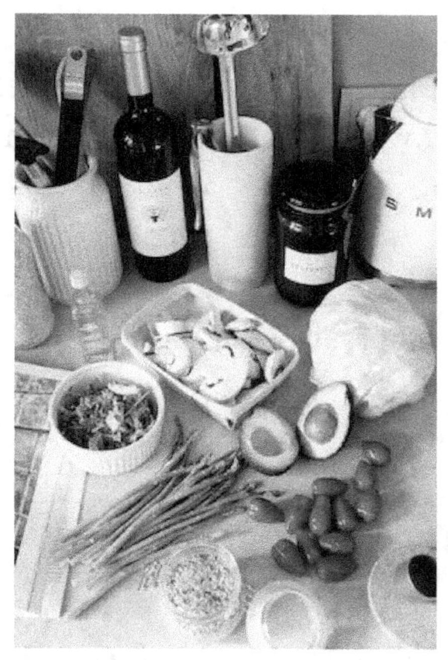

Ingredients:

- 1 medium tomato, diced;
- 1 ripe avocado, peeled and pitted;
- 1/4 cup chopped fresh cilantro; and
- 1 tablespoon of lime juice.
- To taste, salt and pepper

Instructions:

- Blend or process the avocado, tomato, cilantro, lime juice, salt, and pepper until they are completely smooth.

- Place the mixture in a tiny serving bowl, cover it, and serve it cold as a light snack or starter.

Note: To add a spicy kick to this recipe, add diced onion, jalapenos, or hot sauce.

4. *Recipe For Sweet Potato And Apple Puree*

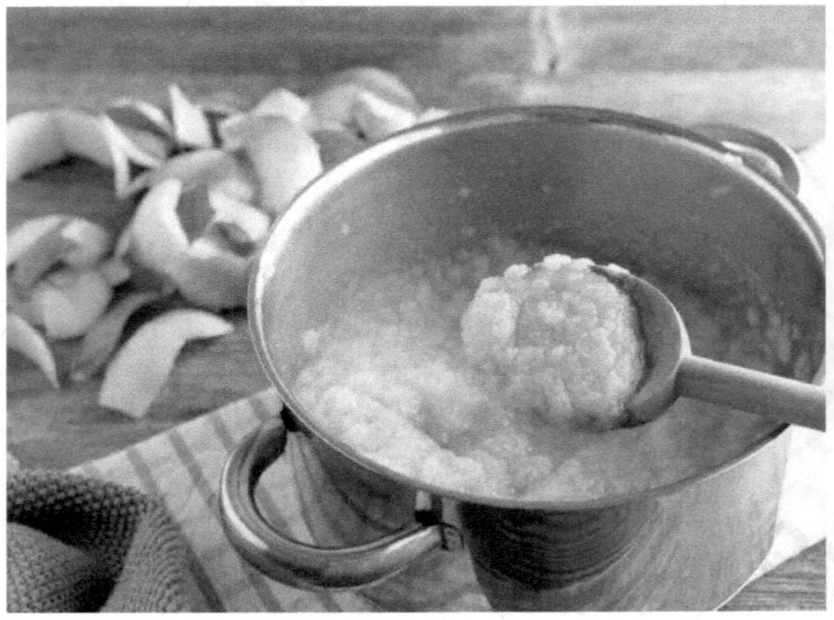

Ingredients:

- 1/4 cup low-sodium chicken broth,

- 1/4 teaspoon ground cinnamon,
- 1 large sweet potato, peeled and diced,
- 1 large apple, peeled and chopped.
- 1/8 teaspoon freshly grated nutmeg
- To taste, salt and pepper

Instructions:

- Combine the sweet potato, apple, chicken broth, cinnamon, nutmeg, salt, and pepper in a medium saucepan.

- Over medium heat, bring the mixture to a boil. Once the sweet potato and apple are cooked through, lower the heat to low and let the mixture simmer for 10 to 15 minutes.

- Pour the mixture into a food processor or blender, and puree until smooth.

- Warm up and serve as a filling side dish or dessert.

Note: You can alter this recipe by switching out the apples or sweet potatoes, or by adding a splash of milk or cream for a creamier texture.

5. *Recipe For Chicken And Vegetable Puree*

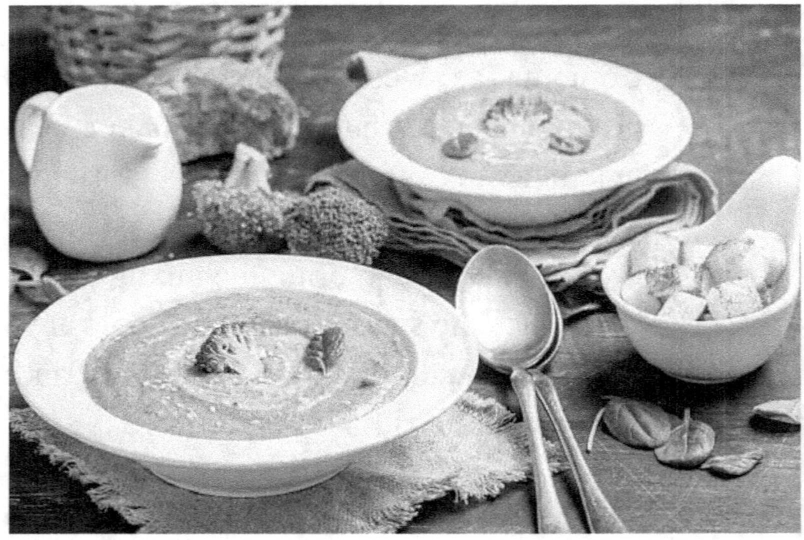

Ingredients:

- 1 boneless, skinless chicken breast is included in the recipe.
- 1/2 medium zucchini, chopped;
- 1 medium carrot, peeled and chopped;
- 1/4 cup low-sodium chicken broth;
- 1 tablespoon olive oil.

-   1 minced garlic clove - Salt and pepper, as desired

Instructions:

- Place a medium saucepan over medium heat and warm the olive oil. When aromatic, add the minced garlic and stir for one to two minutes.

- Add the chicken breast to the pan and cook for four to five minutes on each side, or until browned and well cooked.

- Take the chicken out of the skillet and place it aside. The carrot and zucchini should be chopped, and they should be cooked for two to three minutes in the same pan.

- Stir in the chicken broth and bring the dish to a boil. Once the liquid has been reduced and the vegetables are tender, lower the heat to low and simmer for 5-7 minutes.

- Insert the chicken and vegetables into a food processor or blender, and purée until completely smooth. If more liquid or chicken broth is required to reach the appropriate consistency, do so.

- You can either serve this soup chilled or warm as a main meal.

Note: You can change this dish by including more vegetables like peas, sweet potatoes, or broccoli.

6. *Recipe For Mango And Banana Puree*

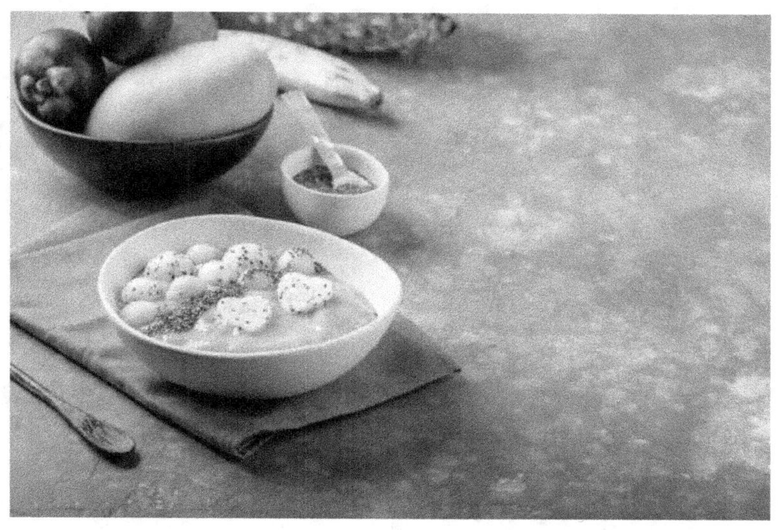

Ingredients:

- 1/4 cup unsweetened coconut milk,
- 1 ripe mango, diced and peeled,
- 1 ripe banana, peeled and sliced.
- 1/4 teaspoon each of ground ginger and cinnamon
- 1 teaspoon of honey

Instructions:

- Puree the mango, banana, coconut milk, ginger, cinnamon, and honey in a blender or food processor until smooth.

- Pour the mixture into a small serving bowl, cover, and chill in the fridge for at least 30 minutes.

- To make a healthy and energizing dessert or snack, serve it cold.

Remark: You can alter this recipe by including more tropical fruits like pineapple or papaya and modifying the honey amount to tataste

- Recipes For Special Diets (Such As Gluten-free, Low-sodium, Etc.)

Here are some recipes for special diets that are appropriate for seniors with dietary restrictions:

1. Chicken And Rice Casserole Without Gluten

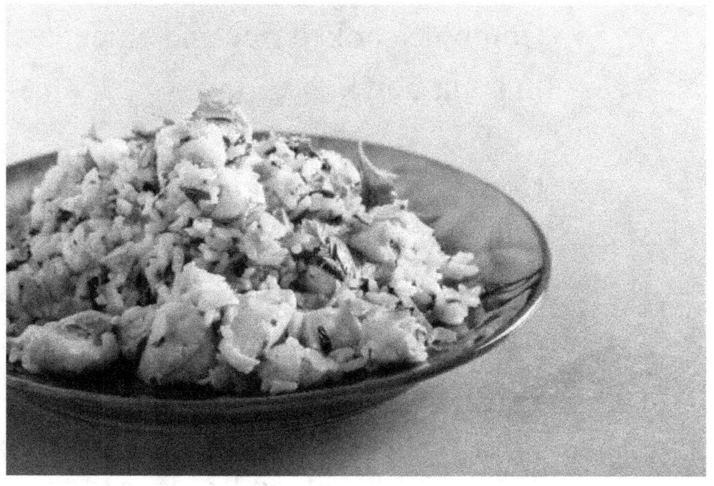

Ingredients:

- 2 cups cooked rice,

- 1 pound cooked and shredded boneless, skinless chicken breast.
- One (10.5 oz) can of condensed chicken soup
- A cup of milk
- A half-cup of gluten-free breadcrumbs
- 1/4 cup melted butter - 1/2 cup finely grated Parmesan cheese
- To taste, salt and pepper

Instructions:

- Set the oven to 350 degrees Fahrenheit.

- Combine cooked rice and chicken shreds in a big bowl.

- Combine the cream of chicken soup and milk thoroughly in another basin.

- Add the soup mixture to the rice and chicken, stirring to combine.

- To taste, add salt and pepper to the food.

- Pour the mixture into a baking dish that measures 9 x 13 inches.

- Combine the melted butter, Parmesan cheese, and gluten-free breadcrumbs in a small bowl and stir until crumbled.

- Cover the casserole's top evenly with the breadcrumb mixture.

- Bake for 30-35 minutes, or until bubbling and golden brown.

2. *Sodium-Free Beef Stew*

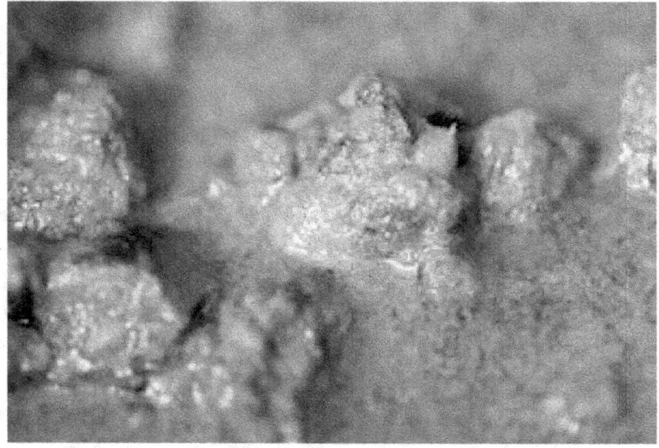

Ingredients:

- 1 pound of beef stew meat, diced into bite-sized pieces.
- 1 tablespoon olive oil
- 1 chopped onion
- 2 minced garlic cloves
- 3 sliced and peeled carrots
- 3 cut celery stalks
- 3 chopped and peeled potatoes
- 1 tsp dried thyme - 1 tsp dried rosemary - 4 cups low-sodium beef broth
- To taste, salt and pepper

Instructions:

- In a large pot over medium-high heat, warm the olive oil.

- Add the beef stew meat and heat for 5 minutes, or until browned on all sides.

- Include the onion and garlic in the pot and cook for 3 minutes or until tender.

- Add the potatoes, carrots, and celery to the pot and stir everything together.

- Add the thyme, rosemary, salt, and pepper to the pot with the beef broth.

- Bring the mixture to a boil, then lower the heat to a simmer, cover, and cook for an hour, or until the meat is thoroughly cooked.

3. *No-Sugar Apple Crisp*

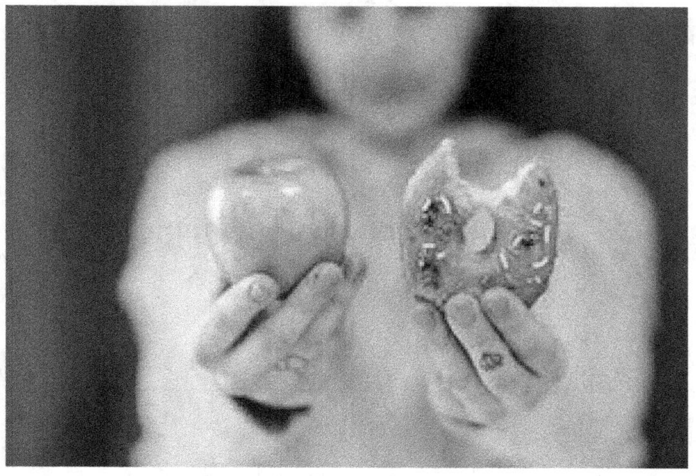

Ingredients:

- sixteen cups of sliced and peeled apples;
- one-half cup of all-purpose flour;
- one-half cup of quick-cooking oats;

- one-half cup of chopped walnuts;
- one-half cup of unsweetened applesauce;
- one-fourth cup of melted butter.
- 2 tsp. cinnamon
- 1/4 tsp salt
- 1/2 tsp nutmeg

Instructions:

- Set the oven to 350 degrees Fahrenheit.

- Combine the flour, oats, walnuts, cinnamon, nutmeg, and salt in a sizable basin.

- Add the melted butter and applesauce to the bowl and stir to incorporate.

- Add the apple slices and stir.

- Pour the mixture into a baking dish that measures 9 x 13 inches.

- Bake the topping for 30-35 minutes, or until it is golden brown and the apples are soft.

4. Chicken And Vegetable Puree Without Gluten

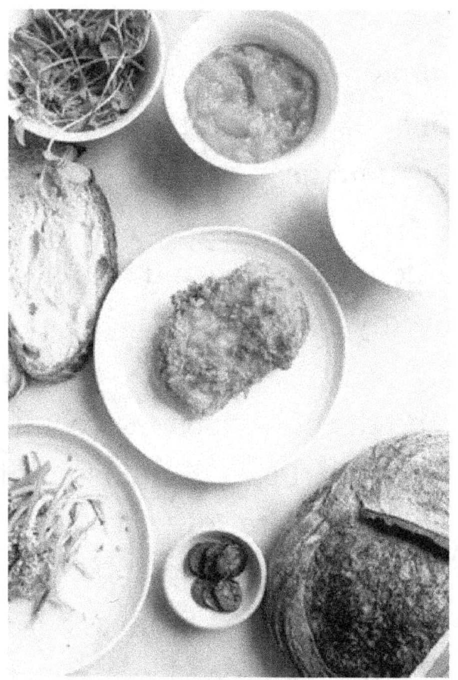

Ingredients:

- 1 pound of cubed boneless chicken breast
- 1 large, peeled, and chopped carrot
- 1/2 sliced zucchini

- Chopped half a red bell pepper
- 1/2 chopped onion
- 2 minced garlic cloves
- 2 cups of chicken broth
- 1 tablespoon of olive oil
- To taste, salt and pepper

Instructions:

- In a big pot, heat the olive oil over medium heat.

- Add the chicken and heat it until it is evenly browned.

- Add the bell pepper, zucchini, carrot, onion, garlic, and sauté until the vegetables are soft.

- Add the chicken broth and heat through. Simmer for around 20 minutes on low heat.

- Using a blender or food processor, puree the ingredients until it is smooth.

- To taste, add salt and pepper to the dish.

5. *Sweet Potato And Carrot Puree With Low Sodium:*

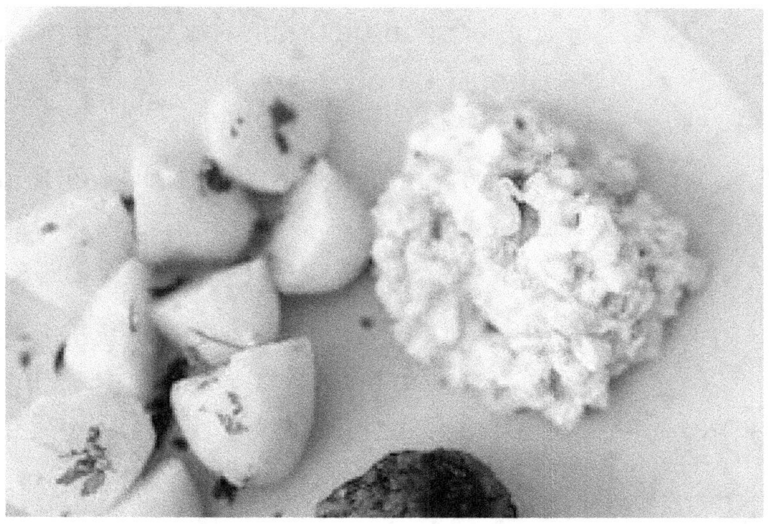

Ingredients:

- Two large sweet potatoes, peeled and chopped;
- Two large carrots, peeled and chopped;
- Two cups of low-sodium chicken broth;
- one-half teaspoon of cinnamon.
- 1/4 teaspoon nutmeg
- To taste, salt and pepper

Instructions:

- Bring the sweet potatoes, carrots, and chicken stock to a boil in a large pot. When the vegetables are ready, turn down the heat and let the mixture simmer for about 20 minutes.

- After draining, save the cooking liquid for later use.

- In a blender or food processor, puree the veggies until they are smooth, adding a little of the leftover cooking liquid at a time to get the right consistency.

- Season with salt, pepper, nutmeg, and cinnamon.

6. *Puree Lentils And Spinach For Vegetarians:*

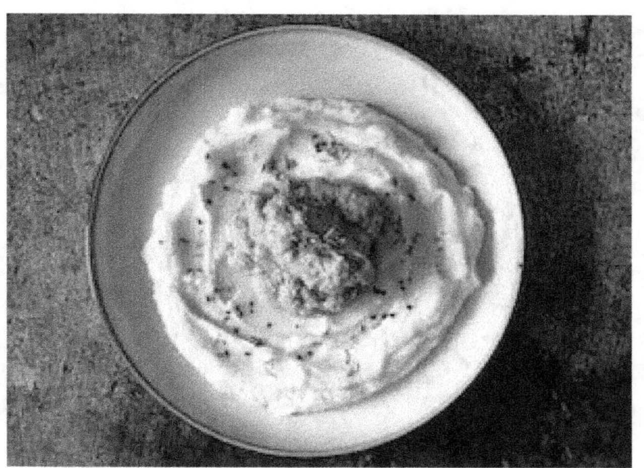

Ingredients:

- 3 cups vegetable broth,
- 1 cup red lentils,
- 1/2 chopped onion.
- 2 minced garlic cloves
- 2 cups chopped spinach
- 1 tablespoon olive oil
- To taste, salt and pepper

Instructions:

- Drain the lentils after giving them a cold water rinse.

- In a big pot over medium heat, warm the olive oil. Sauté the garlic and onion together until the onion is soft.

- Fill the saucepan with the lentils and vegetable stock, then heat to a boil. Once the lentils are ready, turn down the heat and let the mixture simmer for about 20 minutes.

- Stir in the chopped spinach and simmer for a further five minutes.
- Use a blender or food processor to puree the ingredients until it is smooth. To taste, add salt and pepper to the dish.

Note: Depending on specific dietary demands and restrictions, these recipes may need to be modified. They should only be used as broad guidelines. Before making major dietary adjustments for a senior, it is usually prudent to seek advice from a medical practitioner or certified dietitian.

Chapter 5: Planning And Storing Meals

- Advice On Meal Preparation

Here are some suggestions for meal preparation when preparing pureed foods for older people:

- To ascertain the person's unique dietary requirements, speak with a medical expert or a licensed dietitian.

- To maintain a balanced and varied diet, schedule meals in advance and make a weekly plan.

- Prepare meals that have been pureed in larger amounts and freeze them in portions for later use.

- To make meals more tasty and nourishing, use seasonal foods.

- To avoid boredom and retain an interest in eating, use a variety of textures and flavors.

- Instead of using salt, think about utilizing herbs and spices to flavor food.

- Use a range of protein-rich foods, such as tofu, beans, fish, eggs, and poultry.

- To add diversity to the dishes, experiment with various cooking techniques like roasting, grilling, and steaming.

- To make meals interesting and pleasurable, be inventive and test out new recipes and ingredients.

- When planning meals, keep in mind any dietary restrictions or intolerances and make any required adjustments.

- Consider any physical restrictions the person may have, such as trouble swallowing or chewing, and modify the food's texture as necessary.

- To supply important vitamins and minerals, including a variety of colorful fruits and vegetables in your diet.

- Use fortified foods or supplements to make sure you're getting enough nutrients.

- Use healthy fats to enhance flavor and encourage satiety, such as avocado or olive oil.

- Don't forget to stay hydrated; drink plenty of water and other liquids throughout the day, and think about including pureed water-rich fruits and vegetables like watermelon and cucumber.

- To acquire their feedback and raise their involvement with food, think about incorporating the person in the meal planning process.

These suggestions can help you make sure that pureed meals are pleasant and nutritious while also being adapted to the individual's needs and preferences. 11. Consider any physical restrictions the person may have, such as trouble swallowing or chewing, and modify the food's texture as necessary.

- Serving Guidelines And Portion Sizes

Depending on the person's unique dietary requirements and preferences, portion sizes may change while providing pureed meals. The following are some general principles to bear in mind:

To discover the proper portion sizes for a person's unique nutritional requirements, speak with a medical practitioner or nutritionist.

To guarantee uniformity in amount proportions, think about utilizing measuring cups or portion-control containers.

Before serving, be sure that meals that are served hot have reached a safe temperature.

Before serving, be sure that cold meals or snacks have reached a safe temperature.

Make the meals more enticing by using decorative and eye-catching serving utensils.

To improve the meal's flavor and presentation, think about adding garnishes or toppers.

To encourage a happy dining experience, provide food in a cozy and soothing setting.

Keep in mind that the objective is to make eating time joyful and nourishing for the person. You can ensure that someone is getting the nutrition they need while still enjoying their meals by keeping portion sizes reasonable and taking into account the individual's preferences.

- Storage And Reheating Techniques

When it comes to pureed meals, proper storage, and reheating are crucial factors to take into account, particularly for seniors who may have compromised immune systems or other health issues. Observe the following advice:

Pureed food should be kept in the freezer or refrigerator in airtight containers. To keep track of what is inside, use clear containers or label them with the date and contents.

Meals should be refrigerated as soon as they are finished cooking, ideally within two hours. A meal should be thrown away if it was kept at room temperature for longer than two hours.

Use a microwave or a stovetop to cook the food to a safe temperature of at least 165°F (74°C) before reheating.

To achieve consistent heating, stir the pureed food before reheating.

Before reheating the pureed food, think about adding a tiny amount of liquid (such as water or broth) to keep it from drying up.

To avoid splatters when reheating in the microwave, cover the container loosely with a lid or paper towel.

Pureed foods shouldn't be heated up more than once. Reheated leftovers should be kept in the freezer or refrigerator.

The risk of foodborne disease can be decreased and elders can receive nourishing and pleasant meals by ensuring that pureed meals are kept and reheated securely.

Chapter 6: Final Verdict

- Key Points

Key Ideas

For seniors who have trouble chewing or swallowing, pureed food is crucial because it offers a secure and convenient approach to acquiring essential nutrients.

Because homemade pureed food can be customized, fresh ingredients may be used, and the texture and seasoning can be more precisely controlled.

There are several kinds of pureed food, such as fine, coarse, and mechanically soft, and various adjustments can be made to satisfy varied nutritional needs.

A blender, food processor, and strainer are necessary kitchen appliances for pureeing, and for some recipes, specialist tools like a hand-held immersion blender or potato ricer can be helpful.

Both taste and nutrition depend on using fresh, high-quality ingredients.

For pureed meals, cooking methods like roasting, boiling, or steaming can be utilized, and seasoning and flavoring are crucial for improving taste.

A balanced and diverse diet can be ensured with the help of meal planning and quantity control.

To avoid contamination and preserve quality, proper storage, and reheating are essential.

Caretakers and family members can make sure that their elderly loved ones are receiving nourishing and delectable pureed meals that suit their dietary needs and preferences by adhering to these recommendations.

In conclusion, pureed food is a crucial dietary choice for seniors who have trouble swallowing or chewing solid meals. Homemade pureed food is a healthy and inexpensive substitute for store-bought items. Pureed meals can be delectable and filling if fresh ingredients, the right cooking methods, and the right seasoning and flavoring are used. A balanced diet for seniors can be provided by meal planning and portion control, as well as specialized equipment that can make the process simpler. The quality and safety of pureed food can be maintained with proper storage and reheating. Caretakers and family members can provide elders with wholesome, scrumptious pureed meals that support their health and welfare by using these suggestions and recipes.

- Importance Of Serving Seniors Nutritious Pureed Meals

Seniors should be given nourishing pureed meals for a variety of reasons. First off, by ensuring they get the nutrients they require to stay healthy, it aids to preserve their general health and well-being. Seniors may experience decreased appetite or swallowing issues, which, if untreated, can result in malnutrition. Meals that have been pureed are a fantastic approach to giving kids the nutrition they require.

Second, pureed foods can aid in avoiding issues caused by difficulties swallowing. Seniors who have trouble swallowing whole foods run the risk of choking or aspiration, which can result in life-threatening conditions including pneumonia. Caregivers can help lower the possibility of these issues and keep seniors safe by serving pureed meals.

Last but not least, feeding seniors nourishing pureed meals can significantly enhance their quality of life. Eating is a significant social activity in addition to being a means of obtaining essential nutrients. elders can find comfort and delight in sharing meals with others, and pureed meals that are enticing and savory can make elderly feel more included in social situations.

Overall, it's crucial to serve elders wholesome pureed meals for their wellbeing, security, and standard of living.

Review:

We sincerely hope that you have liked our pureed food and first-rate service. We are constantly working to give our customers the greatest experience possible, and we would sincerely appreciate any comments you may have. We would appreciate it if you could take the time to post a review on our website or social media platforms. Your frank comments will enable us to enhance our services and guarantee that we continue to satisfy your demands.

We appreciate your ongoing assistance.

best wishes

Chef Vita

9 798393 966102